*This is the book [...] sending to you in it[...] report (one of many) [...] was aware of the fact that Vit C cures cancer, but dragged their feet about publicizing this.*

# Ridiculous Dietary Allowance

*One of the arguments given is that no animal studies have been done to prove this. I guess it ignores the idea that we are animals.*

## An open challenge to the RDA for vitamin C

*A dose of 60 grams given IV (that's 60000 mg) 3 times a week will arrest and/or kill solid tumors.*

**by**

*Love*
*Gordon*

**Dr Steve Hickey**

**and**

**Dr Hilary Roberts**

# Preface

In recent years, there has been a controversy around Vitamin C's contribution to health. Our aim in this book is to reveal the flaws in the research underlying the recommended dietary allowance (RDA) for vitamin C, in the United States and United Kingdom. Various RDA values are purported to specify the minimum intake required for good health in different sections of the population, such as young children or the aged. For simplicity, we consider mainly the recommended intake for young adults. The RDA has been renamed Dietary Reference Value (DRV) in the UK since 1991. The UK government committees separated the RDA into several subsidiary values, claiming it had been used incorrectly to assess individual diets. The values are the estimated average requirement (EAR), reference nutrient intake (RNI), lower reference nutrient intake (LRNI) and safe intake (SI). A similar subdivision has occurred in the US RDA values, provided by the Institute of Medicine. The Food and Drug Administration had their own version of the RDA[A] for food labelling, based on the Institute of Medicine values; this term has now been changed to Dietary Reference Intake. The renaming and subdivision of RDA values is not pertinent to our discussion.

We first came across the title, "Ridiculous Dietary Allowance", as a description of the RDA by Dr Ron Hunninghake. We thought the phrase was apt, so we borrowed it for our title. There are many derivatives, such as "Ridiculous Dietary Arbitrary". The common use of these slightly derogatory phrases by nutritional scientists indicates the disdain they feel for the RDA concept and its official implementation.

Most of the references are to the recommendations of the Food and Nutrition Board of the US Institute of Medicine. We describe the Food and Nutrition Board as "the committee" throughout. The book also covers the information provided as justification for the upper limits on intake by the Expert Group on Vitamins and Minerals (EVM) of the Food Standards Agency

---

[A] The FDA RDA is sometimes called the U.S. RDA but we use the term US RDA to differentiate the US from the UK recommendations.

in the UK.[1,2,3,4] We generally refer to the EVM as the UK committee, the expert committee or occasionally the committee. While the remit of the EVM was for determining the upper limit, much of their discussion relates to recommended intakes. This book covers the faulty science supporting Tolerable Upper Limits and the other nutritional measures associated with the RDA. The UK RDA in was actually determined in 1991 by the Committee of Medical Aspects of Food and Nutrition Policy (COMA),[5] this committee has now been replaced by the Scientific Advisory Committee on Nutrition (SACN). Review of the dietary reference values for nutrients has been discussed by SACN but there is no timescale for actually carrying out this work.[B,6] We therefore concentrate on the justification for the US RDA, as this essentially encompasses that of the UK recommendations and presents generally higher values. The recent work of the UK EVM on tolerable upper limits is included, as it links closely with the underpinnings of the Codex Alimentarius. While there are differences in the published accounts, the gross errors are consistent. The published justifications do not represent a cost benefit analysis and are selectively biased towards acceptance of low doses.

The evidence used to support the US RDA is published elsewhere,[7,8] and to avoid repetition we often refer to facts in these documents without specifically enumerating the reference. The justification for the RDA is essentially a review of a selected proportion of the available literature. We have often referred to the RDA documents rather than the source papers, specifying the original papers where necessary. The references are provided as sources of additional information, as opposed to specific validation. We recommend readers who are interested in following the chain of evidence to examine the published RDA justifications, which are available online.

This book follows the publication of *"Ascorbate: The Science of Vitamin C"*[9] by the same authors. The *Ascorbate* book provides a synthesis of the current science on vitamin C and presents some new ideas, including the dynamic flow model. In the process, it brings into focus the ideas and experimental basis underlying the

---

B A search of the SACN website found no results for "vitamin C".

RDA. Since this account is supplementary to the *Ascorbate* book, the original references and full arguments are not presented here. Interested readers are encouraged to examine the background in more detail in the original book.

In the present book, we assume that readers have a reasonable appreciation of the number of diseases vitamin C is claimed to prevent or treat, and the magnitude of the effect. Linus Pauling has described the potential health benefits of high doses of vitamin C, in his book *How to Live Longer and Feel Better*.[10] Numerous other books and publications exist, but Pauling's simple writing style and wonderful grasp of his subject make his books classics in this area. A reasonably full account of the pharmacology and medical uses of high doses of vitamin C has been provided by Dr Tom Levy, in his excellent book "Vitamin C, Infectious Diseases and Toxins".[11] We recommend this book to anyone interested in the use of high-dose ascorbate in treating disease.

We have cited several papers by the NIH ascorbate pharmacokinetic group and associated researchers. In referencing these and related papers, we are explicitly not making a statement about the accuracy or validity of any part of this research. In the future, it may be necessary for us to illustrate further errors in these papers. The standard of the science used to support the RDA is, at best, suspect.

In the text, we describe a simple, qualitative, cost-benefit analysis. We are aware that this approach generally applies to quantitative or quasi-quantitative methods. Our aim is simply to indicate that formal decision support theory[12,13] would prevent the bias that is apparent in the current RDA and Tolerable Upper Limit recommendations. We have used the decision analysis terms in a loose way, consistent with a basic description. Our presentation has been simplified to draw attention to the arbitrary nature of the decision making process associated with the RDA for vitamin C and other nutrients. Describing the method in this qualitative way makes it easier to understand, while allowing a structured approach to the decision making process.

The gross limitations in the methods employed in the RDA and upper limits for vitamin C are also found in the recommendations for other nutrients. In particular, we note that the current Codex Alimentarius proposals, based on Tolerable Upper Limits, lack scientific support and may result in innumerable cases of chronic disease and death.

We have tried to be accurate in this book while simplifying the arguments for the non-specialist reader. This balance involves a compromise and readers should feel free to report any errors found in this text to radicalascorbate@yahoo.com.

# Acknowledgements

We would like to thank Bill Sardi, for his magnificent efforts in publicising the challenge to the RDA. Bill is a medical journalist who claims to be a layman, although his knowledge of nutrition exceeds that of many specialists.

Owen Fonorow of the Vitamin C Foundation was the original champion of the dynamic flow model. We greatly appreciate his work in making the claims for vitamin C known to the public.

We would also like to thank the other experts who signed the letter requesting a re-evaluation of the RDA for ascorbate: Professor Ian Brighthope, Robert F. Cathcart III, MD, Abram Hoffer, MD, PhD, FRCP, Patrick Holford, Archie Kalokerinos, MD, Thomas Edward Levy, MD, JD, Richard A. Passwater, PhD, Hugh D. Riordan, MD, and Andrew W. Saul, PhD.

Dr Balz Frei of the Linus Pauling Institute helped us by mounting a private defence of the RDA. His openness on the topic has been refreshing, when compared with the unscientific lack of communication from many establishment scientists.

Dr David Lidbury, of the Institute of Optimum Nutrition, read the text for scientific content and provided many helpful comments. Dr Lidbury is currently working on a project with Patrick Holford on the rational evaluation of nutrient intakes.

Optometrist Dr Sydney Bush provided helpful feedback and discussion of "CardioRetinometry", a technique he proposes for the determination of scurvy. Dr Bush kindly provided information about his definition of scurvy in relation to retinal blood vessel damage and the sample images presented. Quentin Bush also helped and discovered retinal images showing changes in cholesterol.

Dr Peter Keen provided feedback on the initial version of this book. Holly Matthies, Andrew Hickey, Pauline Rose and Gillian Perkins read the manuscript for errors and checked references. Billie Fonorow provided help with editing and checked parts of the manuscript for errors.

Dedicated to Bill Sardi,

for his outstanding work in health and communication.

# Introduction

By Owen Fonorow, Co-founder, The Vitamin C Foundation

In 1920 British biochemist Jack Cecil Drummond suggested that the antiscurvy factor in food, in the absence of chemical information as to the nature of the factor, be named "vitamin C." Other vitamins had been isolated and were found to be coenzymes, somewhat complicated substances that are required for life in small amounts in order to make the enzymes work properly. Nature, in its efficiency, provided these necessary substances in food because they would be difficult for human cells to manufacture; they occur in sufficient amounts in the ordinary diet. When these molecules are missing, a deficiency-disease results.

Vitamin C was the exception to the vitamin rules almost from the beginning. Like the other vitamins, small amounts were observed to have powerful effects on those suffering from a deficiency-disease. Unlike other vitamins, which had few effects in healthy people taking more than an ordinary small amount of a vitamin, vitamin C was found to cure diseases other than scurvy when given in high amounts.

The fragile substance was hard to isolate and was one of the last vitamins whose chemical nature was understood. Given the technical name ascorbic acid, it was found that vitamin C had a sugar-like molecular structure. Later, it was determined that ascorbic acid is not a vitamin necessary in the diet for the vast majority of animal species, most of which make large quantities in their kidneys or livers.

In 1934, shortly after synthetic vitamin C became available, the medical world published the vitamin's unexpected successes in disease-curing and prevention. Professor A. Szent-Gyorgyi, the Hungarian chemist who played a major role in the artificial manufacture of this vitamin, stated that "These curative effects suggest that humanity is suffering much more gravely from a lack of vitamin C than has hitherto been supposed."

Aware of these early findings regarding ascorbic acid, Linus Pauling wrote in 1986 that "Vitamin C has been under investigation, reported in thousands of scientific papers ever since it was discovered (circa) fifty years ago. Physicians had observed at that time that amounts of vitamin C of a hundred to a thousand times larger (than the RDA) have value in controlling various diseases."

American biochemist Irwin Stone, the scientist who first brought the values of ascorbic acid in excess of the RDA to Linus Pauling's attention in the late 1960s, had long argued that vitamin C had been misnamed a "vitamin". Stone felt the name implied that the substance is only required in tiny amounts, and urged instead that it be called the "missing stress hormone" or simply ascorbate. Vitamin C may behave as a coenzyme in conditions that help control scurvy, but its molecular structure is unlike that of other (complicated) coenzymes. Vitamin C as ascorbic acid is derived from glucose in other plants and animals that manufacture it. Also, it shares with glucose many of the same mechanisms for entering and feeding of cells, including insulin-mediated transport into cells.

Thanks to Linus Pauling, we know that super health can be attained by simply taking a few of certain pills daily, emphasizing ascorbic acid. Children are no exception. The following is a personal story that I believe demonstrates, first hand, the effectiveness of vitamin C when taken even before birth. In 1989, following the advice of American physician, Fred Klenner, MD, and after receiving the endorsement of Linus Pauling, my wife and I, before conception, provided our son with high amounts of vitamin C. She continued with 9,000mg daily during pregnancy and more during lactation (10 grams). Our son has ingested multiple grams of ascorbic acid from early infancy, and continues to do so at age 14. He's average height and lean, exceeds the performance of athletes in his physical fitness testing, and has had continuous unusually good health. He's never had an ear infection that "every child" supposedly gets, and the only childhood illness he's had was a mild case of chicken pox. There is no doubt in our minds that these positives in our son's life, are, in great part, due to his taking Vitamin C. He supplements at least 6,000mg of vitamin C daily, with added antioxidants vitamin A, E, B-complex and as complete a multiple vitamin/mineral as possible. This is the regimen described in Linus Pauling's book, "How to Live Longer and Feel Better". All parents deserve the joy of an optimally healthy child and it is easy.

I have often made the statement to our son that although he has been ill, he has never really felt sick a day in his life. Once, when he questioned our assessment that he had never really felt ill, I asked him if he'd like to stop the vitamin C for a while and perhaps experience illness as others do. He declined. I now attribute feeling ill, generally, to the vitamin C depletion caused by fighting the disease. A similar effect causes the hangover after alcohol intake, which can be completely avoided by high dose vitamin C intake.

The Vitamin C Foundation recommends that everyone supplement 3000mg ascorbic acid daily. With the knowledge of Dynamic Flow provided by Drs. Hickey and Roberts, we now suggest spacing that amount throughout the day, perhaps 1,000 mg with every meal. Note: this is our minimum daily allowance. Our recommendation is more that 30 times that of the U. S. Government's National Academy of Sciences. (75-90mg) and 15 times more than that of the current Linus Pauling Institute and Levine's group at the National Institutes of Health (200mg).

Linus Pauling himself prescribed 2 to 6 times the Foundation's vitamin C RDA (6,000 to 18,000mg of vitamin C). Pauling wrote that his dosage was based on the large amounts of vitamin C that animals' bodies manufacture to achieve similar levels.

Vitamin C author/expert Thomas E. Levy, MD, JD, advises from 2 to 4 times our recommendation (6,000 to 12,000mg daily). Our suggestions are based partly on the work of Dr. Robert Cathcart, who determined that the ability to tolerate oral intakes of the vitamin varies between 4 and 16 grams daily, during ordinary (not severe) poor health. Cathcart's clinical experience demonstrates that almost all human beings will tolerate 4 grams of vitamin C daily.

The Vitamin C Foundation advocates 1 gram vitamin C daily for children, based upon their age, up to the age of 3: 1 gram for 1-yr-olds; 2 grams for 2-yr olds, etc. Our suggested daily allowance may not prevent or resolve such diseases that are related to the lack of vitamin C. For example, we believe that heart disease requires from 6,000 to 18,000mg Vitamin C daily, and that cancer may require 14,000 to 39,000mg daily.

The great unanswered question is why humans evolved differently than most animals. If vitamin C is more than a vitamin, how did the human species, like the guinea pig, fruit bat, and a number of higher level primates, survive after losing the ability to make ascorbic acid? Whatever the reason for our survival, there is little doubt this great deficiency in our genetic makeup, the lost ability to produce the enzyme L-gulonolactone oxidase in our livers, an enzyme that would otherwise allow us to convert ordinary glucose (sugar) into ascorbic acid, is what ultimately causes the major chronic illnesses of humankind.

Oct 2004

# Contents

# Reluctant activists

A scientific debate has raged for decades about the required intakes of vitamin C. The medical establishment have taken the view that we only need a tiny amount. The opposition, led by the outstanding chemist Linus Pauling, claimed that large doses could prevent a host of diseases, including heart disease, stroke, cancer and infections. This debate is of vital importance, since the outcome could influence the health of the whole of humanity.

This book presents an open scientific challenge to the recommended dietary allowance (RDA) for vitamin C. The RDA is the level of intake that governments specify as sufficient for the health of their populations. A short time ago, we published a book called *Ascorbate: The Science of Vitamin C.*[9] Ascorbate and ascorbic acid are alternative chemical names for vitamin C. The *Ascorbate* book contains a description of the scientific evidence concerning the use of vitamin C in health and disease. We did not intend the book to be an assault on the RDA but, in writing it, we became increasingly aware that the evidence for a low dose RDA is flawed.

The RDA$^C$ is defined as

"...the dietary intake level that is sufficient to meet the nutrient requirement of nearly all (97 to 98 percent) healthy individuals in a particular life stage and gender group."[8]

We will show that this statement is unjustified in the case of vitamin C and, by implication, the other nutrients to which similar claims are applied.

In this book, we go further into the justification for the RDA. We show that the government committees do not use appropriate decision making methods. Indeed, we found no evidence that they were even aware of the decision support techniques normally used in scientific optimisation. We suggest that their preconceptions have biased the range of intakes

---

$^C$ There are several definitions of the RDA, not all of which are consistent.

considered. As a direct result, their consideration of the scientific literature was selective and unrepresentative. We can find no evidence for the RDA that can be described as compelling, consistent or even reliable.

The RDA concept takes almost no account of individual variation. From a biological standpoint, this seems an unnecessary limitation. The Food and Nutrition Board in the US was established in 1940 and the first edition of its "Recommended Daily Allowances" was published in 1943. Modern biology is about diversity and professional biologists are aware that variation is at the heart of their subject.[14] Genetic techniques highlight people's uniqueness, and medicine is moving towards tailoring interventions to the individual. Conceptually, the RDA belongs to a bygone age of science, before even the structure of DNA was known. The proposition that everyone in the population has the same daily requirement for vitamin C demands hard evidence, but such evidence does not exist.

In 1996, Dr Mark Levine's research group at the US National Institutes of Health (NIH) published results that appeared to show that the high dose claims of Linus Pauling and others must be invalid. The US RDA values were based upon this work.[15] The group claimed that relatively low doses of vitamin C cause people's blood and tissues to become saturated. If this were true, then higher, gram-level supplements would not be absorbed by our bodies, and would thus have no effect. This idea was in direct conflict with reports claiming that high doses or intravenous levels could cure a variety of diseases.[11]

We approached Mark Levine to find out how they had done their work and whether it was convincing. Initially, he was helpful and went out of his way to make sure we understood the experiments. However, it became clear to us that Levine did not fully comprehend the methods the NIH had used. The work involved a branch of pharmacology called pharmacokinetics, which describes the movement of drugs through the body. Pharmacokinetics relies on biochemical and biophysical principles, which can be misinterpreted. It seemed to us that a misunderstanding had occurred and the NIH papers were flawed.

We explained that it looked as though the NIH had used incorrect methods, and consequentially the results were suspect.

Levine told us that this was a highly technical area and referred our comments to the NIH pharmacokineticist. The pharmacokineticist's reply was that he did not understand our objections! We tried again, but repeated emails yielded little response. Over the following year, the NIH failed to explain the errors in their research. It seemed they had lost interest in communicating with us on this matter.

Exasperated, we contacted the individual members of the Institute of Medicine RDA committee, to see if they could clarify the position. The RDA committee had used the NIH papers in setting their recommendations. This being the case, we hoped they would be willing to explain the NIH data. After reading our objections, would they still hold to the view that the NIH research was solid enough to form the basis of a recommendation for the entire population?

None of the committee members replied, but we did get an official (non-scientific) reply from Dr Linda Meyers, director of the committee. The Institute of Medicine declined the option of explaining how the NIH papers could be interpreted in a way that supported their suggested intakes of vitamin C. They also declined the option of re-evaluating the current RDA values. A re-evaluation would apparently involve reconvening the committee and required funding from external bodies, including the NIH. While they correctly indicated that the NIH should defend their own research, the RDA experts had also misunderstood the results. If the core research supporting the RDA is flawed, confidence in the remaining findings is compromised.

In retrospect, the NIH's stalling should have been expected. However, we were working within the normal scientific rules of engagement. A scientist has an obligation to discuss published results with other researchers. Normally, scientists welcome debate and interest in their work. This is not the case with vitamin C. For several decades, the medical and nutritional establishment have ignored claims for high-dose vitamin C. They claim that their selective view of the evidence is scientific, but it is not.

The establishment group is small, yet holds undue influence. The committees and organisations that specify and validate the government recommended intake of nutrients also control the funding for research in this area. By holding positions of influence, they can prevent funding of high-dose studies. When such studies are presented to a medical or scientific journal, these establishment members often act as referees, who can prevent publication. An example of this suppression is the eight-year delay in publishing a vitamin C cancer trial, described by Ewan Cameron.[16]

The pharmaceutical industry needs sick people, from whom to generate profits. Recently, a medical insider told us that the industry was more interested in treatments than cures. He explained that treatments, especially of chronic disease, produce a continuous income stream. By contrast, a cure is a one-off event. For a cure of a minor illness to be commercially viable, it would need to cost above $25,000 per patient, and much more for a major disease.

The pharmaceutical industry depends on a target population of sick people with financial resources, as found in the western nations. Development of new drugs and treatments is biased towards potential financial rewards. There are many examples of how profits outweigh health as a commercial motive. Profitable cholesterol-lowering drugs are given research funding, rather than malaria treatments for the third world, which would save many more lives. For years, tobacco companies protected their profits, derived from the sale of the drug nicotine, by denying cigarettes were dangerous. In the same way, many people believe the medical industries suppress claims for high dose vitamin C and other nutrients, to protect profits.

International legislation, called the *Codex Alimentarius*, aims to limit the supply of nutritional supplements worldwide. If implemented, the Codex will prevent people from being able to make many of their current health choices. Many independent nutritionists and organisations claim that the aim is to prevent adoption of nutritional supplements that threaten the profits of pharmaceutical companies. Whether or not this is true, the Codex is based on the recommended amounts of nutrients specified by governments.[D] In the UK, many members of the committee

---

[D] The emphasis in the Codex has recently changed to tolerable upper limits or measures of toxicity.

setting the recommendations for upper limits have close financial links to the pharmaceutical industry. The financial interests of the RDA committee in the US are considered confidential and are not disclosed.[E]

## Institutional bias

Linus Pauling, the greatest-ever American scientist, championed the medical and nutritional benefits of high-dose vitamin C until he died in 1994. The medical establishment vilified Pauling, claiming his ideas were nonsense. While he might be a great chemist, they implied, he did not have the necessary background for research in this area. They were wrong. Pauling was a genius of the first order and had already made important medical discoveries. His contribution to biology and medicine was greater than that of any of his critics.

Following Pauling's death, the medical establishment claimed they had solid scientific evidence to show that high doses of vitamin C were not even absorbed into the body.[15,17] They ridiculed Pauling and his followers as new-age proselytisers for a holistic fad.

When we looked at these establishment claims, we found that they had no basis in biology. This is critical. The most important feature of such evidence is that it should be biologically sound. Almost every aspect of the background research that purported to support the RDA was lacking in substance. In addition, we could find no scientific refutation of the claims for high-dose vitamin C. The NIH researchers present themselves as hard-nosed scientists, but appear not to be able to conduct an experiment properly. Likewise, the RDA committee failed to interpret simple scientific data. This is disturbing, as the health of millions depends upon their recommendations.

The medical establishment continues to make outlandish claims for low doses of vitamin C, while refusing to consider genuine scientific questions about high-dose supplementation. The RDA committee explains this approach; in their support for the RDA,[7] they state:

---

[E] Appendices B and C list the current memberships of the RDA committees.

"Data show little increase in plasma steady-state concentrations at intakes [of ascorbate] above 200mg/day."

This statement is simply wrong.[9] Based on the erroneous NIH research, it explains why the establishment believe higher doses are ineffective. As we shall see, the RDA committee assume that the blood plasma of an individual is saturated at a low dose of vitamin C. Ascorbate enters the body by way of the blood stream. If the blood is "saturated", the body tissues can receive no more. Since the committee were convinced that doses above 200mg have no effect, they considered only doses in the range below 200mg for their recommendation. They disregarded higher doses, assuming they are not absorbed into the body. This example illustrates the importance of the NIH results and the bias in the arguments presented for the RDA.

One aim of this book is to clarify these problems. Normally, we would have softened our statements somewhat but the absence of a scientific response from the authorities has left us little choice than to state our objections as clearly as possible. Hence, this book consists of a number of short chapters, dealing with different aspects of the science underlying the current RDA. We have structured the presentation around the use of cost-benefit analysis and the latest understanding of the role of ascorbate in the body. Also, we suggest methods that might be extended to provide direct biophysical measurements for estimating individual requirements.

## Request for revision

The Vitamin C Foundation (www.vitamincfoundation.org), led by Owen Fonorow, followed up our approach to the NIH and US Institute of Medicine by publicising the lack of response. It was clear to the Vitamin C Foundation that something unusual had happened. The establishment experts had been challenged and found wanting. Fonorow has been demanding research into the claims for high doses for many years. Now the scientific basis of the RDA was being questioned, yet the authorities were unwilling or unable to respond.

Bill Sardi, a well-known medical journalist, read the *Ascorbate* book and started a campaign to revise the RDA (www.askbillsardi.com). He sent a written petition to the Institutes of Medicine, Food & Nutrition Board, asking that the RDA be reviewed in the light of new evidence. The letter, signed by leading independent nutritionists and asking for a review of the RDA, is given in Appendix A. Sardi also wrote to US Senator Harkin and the Codex Committee for Dietary Supplements.

Because of these campaigns, what began as a straightforward book about the science of vitamin C catapulted us into the middle of a medical controversy. We had covered some of the ground in the first book, now we decided to take a closer look at how the RDA for vitamin C was justified.

# RDA justification

As stated in the official descriptions,[7,8] the RDA for vitamin C is based on an intake of vitamin C

"that maintains near-maximal neutrophil vitamin C concentrations with minimal urinary loss".

This statement sounds scientific, but that does not mean the concept underlying it is scientifically valid. We need to know what it means, and whether or not it is a sensible way to estimate the vitamin C required by an entire population.

For such an important decision as the RDA, you might think that the researchers would study a large number and variety of subjects, to determine the range of responses in the population. You would be wrong, however. The NIH studies based their estimate on results from just seven healthy, young, male subjects.[F,15] In fact, even this is an overestimate, since more than half of the subjects did not complete the whole set of experiments.

Nonetheless, let us suppose that, by some fluke of nature, these seven young men were a representative sample. Would the method be a logical way to determine the vitamin C needs of the population? The answer is a definite no. The core of the justification is the maintenance of *near-maximal neutrophil vitamin C concentrations*. Neutrophils are a type of white blood cell, which the researchers have chosen to represent the body tissues in general. For the RDA to be valid, neutrophils must be similar to other body cells in their use of vitamin C. However, they are not. White blood cells have unusually high ascorbate requirements, with specialised absorption mechanisms and biochemistry.

On grounds of basic biology, the choice of white blood cells is absurd. White blood cells protect the body by generating oxidants,

---

[F] Fifteen healthy young women were included in a later study by the NIH, which gave similar results.[17]

which they release to destroy bacteria and other foreign bodies. To protect themselves from the free radicals they generate, they need an excess of ascorbate to act as an antioxidant. Neutrophil cell membranes have pumps that can pull ascorbate from surrounding fluids, even when the concentration is low. When asked, Dr Mark Levine indicated that the NIH group chose white blood cells because they were easy to sample. Surprising as it may seem, the RDA committee based their recommendations on the behaviour of these highly specialised white blood cells, despite their obvious differences from other body tissues.

The RDA committee claimed that, in the absence of other data, neutrophils were the *"best* biomarker at the current time"*. The committee did not provide an explanation of how or why they came to this conclusion. The first notable aspect of this claim is the use of the word "best". Scientists do not normally use this word, as it implies a value judgement. Questions arise immediately, regarding the specific way in which neutrophils are considered the "best". Normally, when making a scientific comparison, the relationship is specified. For example, the statement "Fred is better than Susan" is meaningless: Fred might be kinder, cleverer, darker, or any one of a myriad of measures used to make the comparison. If we say, "Fred is better for running the race, because he is faster than Susan", the meaning is clear. When the RDA committee claim that neutrophils are the best biomarker, they are making an unscientific statement.

Even though the RDA committee based their estimate on neutrophil saturation, they chose a sub-saturation value for the RDA. The value the committee recommended was only 80% of the saturated value. This decision to lower the estimate was based on minimising the amount excreted. They suggest this amount provides for adequate antioxidant protection. However, later we will see that they also indicate that protection in activated neutrophils requires high plasma ascorbate levels (284 microM/L[G]). It appears that while carrying out their normal activities, in inflammation and immune response, neutrophils may require higher levels than are normally obtained, even from megadose oral supplementation.

---

[G] The unit "microM/L" is a measure of concentration.

It seems likely that vitamin C requirements vary greatly, both between individuals and within the same individual at different times, depending on state of health. Since the committee did not know the amount of variation, they arbitrarily chose a value of 10%. This figure is not based on evidence. Doubling the number they first thought of, they go on to state that twice this value will be adequate for 97-98% of adults. We cannot comprehend the basis of this calculation; presumably, it uses magical-statistics.[H]

The *Ascorbate* book highlighted the errors in the results on blood plasma, which were gross and misleading. As we will show later, the concept of "minimal urinary loss" is also flawed. The excretion of ascorbate is related directly to plasma concentrations, as is the biochemistry of neutrophils. This book explains how these arguments, used as the basis of the RDA, are unsustainable.

---

[H] We think they assume that the 10 percent variation is the standard deviation. Then they forget they are just guessing, and further assume that by using two standard deviations they have then generated a "statistic" that is valid for 97-98% of the population.

# Cost-benefit analysis

The theory of games developed over about 2000 years. The first known solution to a two-person game[1] was provided by James Waldegrave, in a letter dated 13 November 1713. A notable highlight in the development of the theory was the publication of the "Theory of Games and Economic Behavior" by John von Neumann and Oskar Morgenstern in 1944.[18] Game theory and decision theory provide methods for optimising strategy in decision making.[19,20] Here, we suggest the use of cost-benefit analysis.[21] It is a simple approach, used widely in business, computer science, economics, mathematics, philosophy and political science, but apparently not widely in medicine[22] or nutrition. This has recently been understood by the UK authorities who have included some minor consideration of benefits along with risk in consideration of later nutrition guidelines.[23,24] In the case of nutrition, decision theory could generate optimal guidelines based on rigorous logic.

## The dangers of being over-cautious

The RDA justification documents describe many studies of vitamin C and different diseases.[7,8] The committee's reason for including these is to see whether the studies provide "compelling evidence" to support recommending a particular level of intake. The methods, doses and results of these studies vary greatly, though many of the studies cited suggest vitamin C could be beneficial in preventing disease. Despite this, almost every relevant section concludes with a statement along these lines:

> "Although many of the above studies suggest a protective effect of vitamin C against cardiovascular disease, the data are not consistent or specific enough to estimate a vitamin C requirement based on any of these specific biomarkers for cardiovascular disease".

The phrase that data are *not consistent or specific* enough to estimate the vitamin C requirement occurs several times in the

---

[1] A mixed strategy mini-max solution.

document.[8] It means that if a high dose has an effect, the result is required to be reproducibly confirmed and solid. Based on a comparison with drug trials, this sounds a prudent and conservative approach. However, drugs carry substantial risks and costs: we need to be sure they are effective before exposing people to the dangers. Vitamin C, on the other hand, is an essential nutrient and is extremely safe. If there is even slight evidence that it might be effective against disease, the risks of not taking it could outweigh the costs.

The insistence on data being "consistent and specific" leads almost inevitably to the incorrect recommendation of a low RDA. Suppose there are 10 studies, of which eight show massive benefit and two do not. In this case, the evidence for benefit is not consistent, even if the negative studies indicate no harm, so all the results are discarded. Now, imagine a study shows huge benefits from vitamins C and E, in combination. This would fail the specificity requirement, because ascorbate alone did not produce the effect. The process excludes the established synergy between nutrients, such as vitamin C and vitamin E, from the analysis.

The "consistent and specific" rule preferentially excludes data from high dose studies. This is because there are more studies on low doses (10-200mg), so finding specific, low dose data is easier. Current population intakes are low, so epidemiology adds positive data to support low doses. Data on high doses is relatively sparse, and the filtering method employed by the committee means that a few contradictory results can be used to reject the numerous studies that indicate substantial benefits. Hence, the RDA document repeatedly makes statements such as this:

"Although many of the above studies suggest a protective effect of vitamin C against specific cancers by site, the data are not consistent or specific enough to estimate a vitamin C requirement based on cancer."

This inappropriately high level of apparent caution employed by the RDA committee means that millions of people are being actively discouraged from taking a cheap, harmless supplement that could protect them from cancer, cardiovascular disease and other illnesses. The committee have covertly overestimated the dangers of too much vitamin C, and have grossly underestimated the potential benefits of higher doses.

## Estimating the optimal dose

To determine the optimal dose, it is necessary to use appropriate methods. Cost-benefit analysis is a well-established technique for this sort of problem. Put simply, it weights the benefits against the possible costs:

**Value of dose = Estimated benefit - Estimated harm**

In the case of vitamin C, we consider the probability of a positive effect against the possible toxicity. With this approach, the safety of the substance is compared to the expected benefit. The benefit is the probability of disease reduction or greater health, while the cost is the risk associated with the dose. If the substance is very safe, even a small potential benefit has value. By contrast, if the known harm or toxicity is large, then we would need to demonstrate a large benefit for the dose to be considered valuable.

To take a practical example, the cytotoxic chemotherapy used against some cancers has horrible side effects (cost), but if it saves the person's life (benefit), then it might still be valuable.

**Value of chemotherapy = Chance of saving life - Side effects**

In this case, patients might decide for themselves what value they place on the variables. An old person could think that a slightly extended lifespan is not worth suffering the side effects, whereas a young mother might decide to risk anything, to see her children grow up.[J]

---

[J] Notice here how risk is not the same as probability. Probability is the chance that an event will happen. Risk is the probability of a loss and is therefore a measure of probable harm.

Now let us take another example. Suppose some, but not all, studies suggested the duration of a cold might be decreased by drinking more water.

**Value of drinking more water = Chance of shorter cold - No side effects**

In this case, the cost is approximately zero, so the value is positive, even if the chance of a shorter cold is quite small. There is nothing to lose by drinking a few extra glasses of water if you feel a cold coming on, it will do no harm and might do some good. This low-toxicity example is similar to the situation with vitamin C.

# Recommending a high dose RDA

In order to accept the idea of a higher dose RDA, we need to know that the toxicity of ascorbate is low and that such a dose would be harmless. There are two aspects to this, firstly, high doses of ascorbate must not be acutely toxic and, secondly, they must not cause health problems in the longer term.

If ascorbate were toxic, we would need substantial, reproducible evidence of a large benefit to recommend a high dose RDA. The expected benefit would need to outweigh the expected toxicity. Supposing one in a hundred people developed severe arthritis when supplemented with a gram of ascorbate for 20 years,[K] but the supplement offered a possible reduction in levels of atherosclerosis. We could not recommend a supplement with this level of toxicity, for such a low benefit. However, some benefits could outweigh this level of risk. For example, if high dose vitamin C eliminated atherosclerosis, heart disease and stroke completely, the small risk of developing arthritis would be worth taking.

Balancing the risks against the benefits should be standard practice. For example, the drug paracetamol (acetaminophen) provides minor benefits, such as analgesia and fever relief (antipyretic action). These effects are similar to those of aspirin,

---

[K] Vitamin C supplementation does not cause arthritis.

which works in a similar way. These benefits can be weighed against the drug's high toxicity. Between 1993 and 1997, paracetamol caused up to 500 deaths a year in England and Scotland alone.[25,26] This drug causes about 15% of deaths from poisoning. It is claimed that around 70,000 cases of paracetamol overdose occur annually in Britain.[27] Despite this, about 30 million packs of paracetamol are sold in the UK each year. By way of comparison, the number of reported deaths from poisoning with vitamin C each year is zero. Indeed, we could not find any reported deaths from oral doses of vitamin C at any dose - ever. With such low toxicity, even the suggestion of a minor benefit from ascorbate would dominate a cost benefit analysis.

The strongest reason to reject the option of setting a high dose RDA would be if ascorbate were toxic. Levels of toxicity resulting in death or illness would outweigh all but the most powerful evidence of a beneficial effect of a high dose. In a population of 280 million, such as the United States, even a low expectation of toxicity may be important.

We might also reject a high dose on economic grounds. If ascorbate were expensive, then the cost of supplementation could outweigh a small health benefit. Similarly, if people needed to supplement for many years to achieve the expected benefit, the cost may outweigh the benefits.

### Risks of recommending a high dose RDA

The main problem with recommending an unnecessarily high dose is that toxicity is often dose related. Recommending too high a dose might mean some members of a population suffer side effects. The risk is proportional to the toxicity: if the toxicity is zero, then there is no health risk in taking a large dose. We could accept lower levels of benefit if the health risks of the dose were small.

Since ascorbate appears to be harmless, then even a small potential benefit is valuable. Therefore, a reasonable probability of a minor advantage, such as prevention of the common cold with gram level doses, should be sufficient to validate the recommendation of a high dose RDA.

### Risks of rejecting a high dose RDA

If the committee incorrectly rejects the option of setting a high dose RDA, the population could become undernourished and unhealthy. If high doses are protective against heart disease or cancer, then a large section of the population could suffer if the recommended dose is too low. This risk relates to undervaluing the benefits of higher doses, or overemphasising the toxic effects.

The risk of rejecting a high dose on economic grounds is that the cost of an increase in deficiency diseases could greatly outweigh the money saved. (Of course, those who profit from the treatment of disease might see this as an opportunity, rather than a risk.)

## Recommending a low dose RDA

The presence of toxicity would dictate a recommendation of the lowest dose consistent with the established biological benefits. This scenario corresponds closely to the decision making process undertaken by the RDA committee. They appear to have assumed a minimum dose is always preferable and to have filtered out the evidence supporting higher doses, by requiring "compelling evidence" that is both "consistent" and "specific". Such filters would be appropriate if vitamin C were known to be toxic, which it is not.

### Risks of recommending a low dose RDA

The risk of recommending too low a dose is that the population will be malnourished. Given low toxicity, a low dose recommendation could throw away the benefits of higher doses, for no gain in safety. In the longer term, this might mean that many people would suffer deficiency diseases. With extremely low toxicity, the choice of a low dose is not conservative, unless there is no evidence at all that higher doses offer benefits. Indication of probable benefit at a higher dose would suggest the committee should reject the lower dose recommendation.

### Risk of rejecting a low dose RDA

The major risk of rejecting a low dose recommendation in favour of a higher dose depends on the toxicity. If this is high, then there is a danger of side effects with higher doses. However, if the toxicity is low, these risks are small. Given convincing evidence that the toxicity is low, there would be little need for "compelling evidence" that higher intake values could provide a benefit. Even a small potential benefit would suggest a higher dose could be valuable. In this case, the committee could safely reject a low dose RDA in favour of a higher dose recommendation.

The economic risk of rejecting a low dose recommendation is that people spend more on supplements than they really need. Since ascorbate is cheap, this risk is small.

## RDA decision-making bias

Using the RDA committee's approach, if experiments with high doses show benefits, there must be consistent, supporting evidence. Furthermore, there must be no contradictory data. The committee has applied these rules, regardless of the toxicity. The members presumably intended their approach to be conservative, but it is not.

For each biological indicator, such as atherosclerosis, cancer and so on, the suggestion that the data are not sufficiently compelling, reproducible and specific appears, on face value, to be accurate. However, these requirements are inappropriate. Instead, the committee should ask a series of focussed, cost-benefit questions, to arrive at a justifiable recommendation. For example:

- What benefits do the data suggest?

- What dose was used to achieve this benefit?

- How important is the benefit, relative to the known toxicity at this dose?

Such directed questions would provide a rational evaluation of the data. We will return to the idea that the RDA should be based on a cost-benefit analysis later. Before that, we review the specific arguments used to justify the RDA, starting with prevention of scurvy.

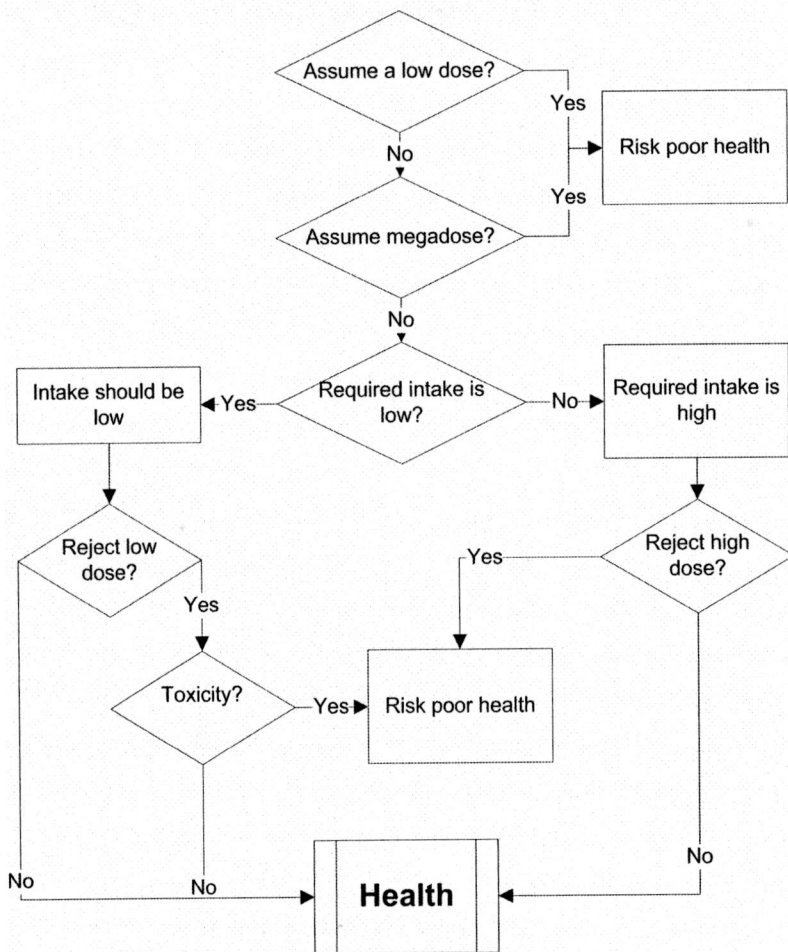

RDA
Risks and bias

Assume a low dose?
No
Yes → Risk poor health
Yes
Assume megadose?
No

Intake should be low ← Yes — Required intake is low? — No → Required intake is high

Reject low dose?
Yes

Reject high dose?
Yes

Toxicity? — Yes → Risk poor health

No    No → **Health** ← No

Flow diagram indicating elements of the decision process.

# Scurvy

People who take insufficient vitamin C over a prolonged period develop scurvy. A person with scurvy is pale, feels depressed, and suffers bleeding from the mucus membranes and into joints, which can make movement difficult or painful. Symptoms include:

- Gum disease

- Weakness

- Joint pain

- Bruised skin

- Corkscrew hairs

Most of the symptoms of scurvy result from an inability to synthesise collagen. Collagen strengthens blood vessels; without it, the body cannot repair damage, and bleeding occurs. It typically takes about three months of vitamin C deprivation for a person to show signs of acute scurvy. Untreated scurvy is fatal. Fortunately, all that is required for an apparently full recovery is to resume intake of a small amount of vitamin C.

Acute scurvy is a severe and dramatic disease. However, it has been suggested that scurvy can also exist in a chronic form. Some scientists believe that if people do not maintain high enough blood ascorbate levels, their bodies cannot repair minor blood vessel damage. In the long term, this leads to atherosclerosis and heart attacks.[28,29,30] Similar suggestions have been made for infection, cancer, arthritis and degenerative brain disease.[31] Later we will describe a new measure of scurvy, which suggests the intake for cardiovascular health should be several grams.

The absolute minimum intake of vitamin C to avoid sickness and death is the amount needed to prevent acute scurvy. Thus, prevention of scurvy indicates a baseline below which the RDA cannot be set. A few milligrams of vitamin C per day prevents acute scurvy in most people. The committee claim that scurvy is associated with a blood plasma level of less than 10 microM/L.

The US RDA committee state that if a person took no vitamin C at all, following a previous daily intake of 75mg, they would not get scurvy for over a month.[8,32] Presumably, we are to assume that this somehow makes a dose of 75mg appropriate. Their statement is quite odd, however, as any adequate intake would have the same effect. We can highlight just how misleading this statement is by quoting from the UK committee justification:

> "If vitamin C is withdrawn from the diet, it takes from 100-160 days for the advanced clinical signs of scurvy to develop." [2]

100-160 days is more than three months. We assume the US committee did not intend to give the impression that an intake of 75mg increases the risk of scurvy, despite suggesting that, at this intake level, scurvy could occur after just one month.

With low intakes of vitamin C, in the range 5-20mg per day, the ratio of oxidised glutathione to reduced glutathione may be increased,[33] indicating oxidative stress. The relative amounts of oxidised and reduced antioxidants, such as glutathione and ascorbate, provide a measure of the health of the organism, at least with respect to redox status.[9]

It is not controversial to suggest that the optimal intake for an individual must be greater than the amount needed to prevent acute scurvy. At these levels, toxicity is irrelevant, as death from scurvy would be worse than any toxic effects. However, most people would agree that prevention of short-term death is an overly conservative choice of criterion for determining the RDA.

# Vitamin C in the body

The RDA committee uses neutrophil white blood cells as a model for normal body tissues. In this section, we show that neutrophils contain far greater amounts of ascorbate than the typical body tissues they are alleged to represent. Neutrophils are also known to have specialised uptake mechanisms, which have not been reported in normal body tissues.

## Body pool

The body pool is the total amount of vitamin C in the body. A body pool below 300mg is associated with scurvy.[34] In a healthy person, the body pool is typically one to two grams.[35]

## Mean concentration in the body

Knowing the body pool, we can estimate an average value for the concentration of ascorbate in the body. To make the numbers easier, consider an adult subject weighing 100kg (220 pounds). We will also assume the subject contains 1.76g ascorbate, which is close to the maximum body pool and is consistent with the mass of the subject.

Given a molecular weight for ascorbate of 176, the concentration of this amount of ascorbate for a volume of one litre (mass one kg) is:

**1.76 / 176 = 0.01 Moles = 10 mM/L**

With a body mass of 100 kg, the average concentration is:

**0.01/100 Moles = 0.1 mM = 100 microM/L**

This figure is slightly higher than the baseline blood plasma level for subjects with good nutrition or supplementation (~70 microM/L).

## Distribution in the Body

This 100 microM/L concentration is an average for the body. However, vitamin C is not evenly distributed. In some tissues, such as adrenals, eyes, brain and white blood cells, the level is much higher and in the millimole per litre range (one mM/L = 1000 microM/L).[36,37,38] Thus, some tissues contain more than ten times the average concentration.[L] These high concentration tissues have a greater requirement, are more sensitive to depletion and absorb more vitamin C from their environment than typical body tissues.[38] The majority of tissues, notably blood plasma and saliva, contain much lower concentrations. Tissues with high levels of ascorbate are atypical, which we can demonstrate using a simple calculation.

To start with, we can estimate how much of the body pool is contained in the specialised tissues. One kg of high concentration tissue, such as brain, at one mM/L contains:

**0.001 x 176 = 0.176g**

The assumption of a concentration of one mM/L is approximate but reasonable.[38,15,17] This is a little less than the concentration in neutrophils and perhaps 20-35% of the value in other white blood cells, monocytes (3 mM/L) and lymphocytes (4 mM/L).

Let us assume that the total mass of this specialised tissue is about 5kg in the body.[M] This approximation is not critical as the value is small relative to the body mass. With these assumptions, we can calculate the mass of ascorbate in the specialised tissues:

**Mass in specialised tissues = 5 * 0.176 = 0.88g**

---

[L] This varied distribution in tissues is recognised by the UK EVM committee.

[M] The known variation in tissue mass and concentration produces similar results.

38

This means that about half the body pool is contained in high concentration in the specialised tissues, which is consistent with the literature.[38]

This localisation of ascorbate implies that the concentration in the majority of the body is lower than the average value for the whole body, as just half the body pool is distributed in about 95% of the body mass. Typical body tissues contain

**100 / (2 x 0.95) = 53 microM/L**

Thus, the concentration in most body cells is of the same order as the baseline blood plasma level (~70 microM/L). This baseline level is a minimum in well-nourished individuals.[9] Most body cells have a concentration that is far lower than the sustained steady state plasma level (~240 microM/L), which can be attained with repeated supplementation.[9,50,38] This suggests that both the body pool and the concentration in normal body tissues could be increased well above currently accepted values, if a sustained steady state were maintained in the plasma.

## Neutrophil concentration

Neutrophils contain far more vitamin C than most other tissues. To illustrate this, suppose we assume that all body tissues behave like neutrophil white blood cells. In this case, the vitamin C body pool for a 100kg human, given an ascorbate concentration within neutrophils of 1.3 mM, would be:

**Body pool = 1.3 * 0.176 * 100 = 23 grams**

This body pool value is at least an order of magnitude (10 times) greater than the maximum estimated body pool. We can therefore reject the idea that these white blood cells are a reasonable model for the body.

The RDA committee claim that neutrophil concentrations correlate well with the body pool. That means that high neutrophil concentrations occur when the body pool is high, and low concentrations when the pool is low. They give a single reference, which suggests more research is needed, to validate this statement.[39] However, it is easy to see how white blood cell concentrations might be related to the body pool. The body pool is the body's store, which protects sensitive tissues from scurvy. When vitamin C is in short supply, tissues such as white blood cells, with large numbers of transporters to absorb ascorbate, deplete slowly and make up the dominant portion of the body pool. However, the majority of tissues in the body are under severe ascorbate shortage during this period, as they deplete more rapidly.

## Ascorbate breakdown

The RDA committee claim that the breakdown rate of ascorbate within the body is 10-45mg per day, over a range of intakes. The committee relate this breakdown level to the body pool size, though they do not provide supporting data or explanations. Presumably, they believe that the breakdown of ascorbate is in some way related to the body's requirements.

Breakdown of ascorbate is unconnected to its known antioxidant functions, which generally involve reversible reactions. When acting as an antioxidant, ascorbate is oxidised to the stable ascorbyl radical or to dehydroascorbate. Oxidised ascorbate is reduced back to ascorbate in an oxidation-reduction cycle. This oxidation-reduction cycle does not involve breakdown of the molecule.

## Concentration of ascorbate transporters

There are two different families of ascorbate transporters, called *sodium dependent vitamin C transporters* (SVCT) and *glucose transporters* (GLUT).[40] These biochemical pumps move ascorbate (SVCT) or dehydroascorbate (GLUT) into cells, and maintain the body pool. It is easy to think that two cells with the same transporter type must be equivalent. However, this assumption is faulty for both body pool and tissue requirements, because the number of transporters varies between cell types. The rate of transport of a particular ascorbate pump (called Km) may be relatively constant across tissues, but the number or concentration of transporters (called Vmax) in the cells is not. A cell with more transporters can pump more vitamin C, and increase its intracellular concentration. By analogy, consider a ship with a hole in its hull. A single pump may not be enough to stop the ship from sinking, but 100 pumps might keep it afloat indefinitely.

The intracellular concentration of ascorbate depends primarily on the number of functioning ascorbate transporters in the outer cell membrane. The RDA committee members have failed to understand the implications of the fact that the concentration of transporters in the outer cell membrane can vary dramatically, for example, in the presence of insulin. This means that estimates of ascorbate "saturation" could be highly glucose dependent.[41] GLUT4[N] transporters are also important for moving glucose into the cell[42,43] and are involved in the mechanism of action of insulin. Variation in insulin levels or blood glucose could directly affect ascorbate levels, particularly within cells.[44,45,46,47] For this reason, the varied blood glucose and insulin levels in the population could invalidate any RDA assumptions based on neutrophils or the body pool. The concentration in many cells could change, as the GLUT4 transporters become saturated (or depleted) with glucose.

The committee accepts that ascorbate concentration varies widely between different body tissues. They indicate that individual tissues have specific transport mechanisms, to allow for this variation. The committee also admits that these transporters vary in type and number, from one tissue to another. The immediate implication of this is that a single cell type would be a poor model to represent all the other tissues in the body.

---

[N] There are several types of glucose transporter which are identified by number. Neutrophils contain GLUT1 and GLUT3, while GLUT4 is insulin sensitive.

# Low dose hypothesis

The word vitamin was derived from "vital amine". Originally, the term was defined as a nitrogenous substance that was required in the diet in small amounts. When scientists discovered that not all such essential factors were amines, they changed the name to vitamin. Nowadays, the term vitamin is often used to mean a micronutrient.

Vitamin C occurs throughout the plant and animal kingdoms. It is a white crystalline substance, also known as ascorbic acid or ascorbate. The name vitamin C was used before it had been isolated as a pure substance. Thus, researchers had classified it as a micronutrient before they even knew what it was. In 1928, Albert Szent-Gyorgyi isolated ascorbate and went on to show it could prevent scurvy: he had identified vitamin C. From this point on, it was possible to carry out proper scientific studies of its properties. However, the name vitamin C stuck, along with the belief that it was a micronutrient.

The idea that dietary ascorbate is required only in small amounts, to prevent scurvy, continued to be the mainstream medical model for the remainder of the 20th century. By the middle of the century, this historical idea had almost the strength of a scientific law. As we have seen, the deficiency disease, scurvy, is prevented by an intake of a few milligrams each day. Most people accepted the definition of ascorbate as a vitamin or micronutrient as obvious.

In scientific terms, however, the idea of ascorbate as a micronutrient is not a law, but a *hypothesis* or proposal to be tested. This is because although ascorbate in small quantities certainly prevents acute scurvy, the *optimal* intake is not established. An intake of 10mg a day from the diet may prevent scurvy, but might not be enough to prevent colds or a chronic disease like arthritis. In order to find the optimal dose, it is necessary to examine a range of intakes. This research has not been done.[9]

The *low dose hypothesis* proposes that ascorbate is a micronutrient, required in trace amounts, and has an associated deficiency disease, called scurvy.

Evidence for the low dose hypothesis might include:

- Showing that scurvy is ascorbate's only deficiency disease

- Showing that prevention of all ascorbate deficiency diseases requires it in micronutrient quantities only

- Showing that measures of "good health" are maximal with low intakes

- Showing that indicators of illness are minimal with low doses

- Showing that higher doses are toxic or in some way deleterious

- Showing that animals with low intakes are more resistant to stress

- Showing that animals with low intakes are more resistant to infection

- Showing that animals with low intakes are more resistant to degenerative disease

- Showing that animals that synthesise ascorbate produce only small amounts

- Since ascorbate is an antioxidant, showing that people are in optimal redox balance with low intakes

- Demonstrating that competing high dose hypotheses are invalid

Other factors could be included in this list. None of these criteria have been demonstrated or have even minimal supporting evidence.

Surprisingly, the most powerful item on this list is the last: demonstrating that the competing high dose hypotheses are invalid. Refutation is more powerful than supporting evidence. The most convincing evidence for the low dose hypothesis would be to show that higher doses are unhelpful, deleterious or even toxic. In proposing a low dose, it is critically important to provide evidence that higher doses are less beneficial.

The health of entire populations depends on the recommendations of the RDA committee. Such huge influence requires a degree of humility and a willingness to consider all the available information. Both scientifically and ethically, recommendation of a low-dose intake requires substantial supporting evidence for the low dose hypothesis. A faulty recommendation could mean that people who follow the advice would be subject to deficiency diseases and premature death.

The current RDA recommendations represent the establishment's estimate of the requirement for vitamin C in humans, based on the low dose hypothesis. We will show that, in their justification for the recommended intake, the committee has assumed the low dose hypothesis to be established before evaluating the data. This assumption leads to a selective view of the available scientific literature, and a potentially biased RDA.

# High dose hypothesis

The high dose hypothesis is the idea that ascorbate is required in doses substantially higher than are needed to prevent scurvy. The actual dose remains to be determined and is likely to vary with the individual and their state of health. However, daily doses in the one to several gram range would fall under this hypothesis. Many people think the high dose hypothesis originated with the chemist Linus Pauling, in the 1960s. In fact, the support for high doses goes back further than this, at least as far as the isolation of ascorbate. Szent-Gyorgyi, who won the Nobel Prize for isolating vitamin C, believed it was a grave error to think that ascorbate was needed only in small amounts. From these early days, he thought the requirement was much larger and in the gram range.

Linus Pauling's name has been closely associated with vitamin C since the 1960s. Irwin Stone, a chemist who had been researching vitamin C since the 1930's, introduced Pauling to the idea of high doses.[48] Stone argued that ascorbate was not a vitamin at all, but was needed in large amounts in the diet. This argument relied on comparison with animals, which manufacture their own vitamin C in their bodies. During evolution, humans lost the ability to make gulonolactone oxidase, one of the enzymes needed to convert the sugar glucose into ascorbate. The situation is more complex than this; for example, some people may retain the ability to manufacture some ascorbate in their bodies.[38] However, this simplified account is adequate for our present purposes.

Most animals synthesise vitamin C and produce it in large quantities. In human terms, these animals seem to synthesise at least gram levels of ascorbate. Dogs, for example, synthesise amounts equivalent to about two and half grams in a human. Many other animals, such as the goat, appear on current evidence to make much more.

Synthesis of ascorbate in gram quantities is not the same as taking these amounts orally. When a healthy person consumes a one gram vitamin C supplement, only a fraction (about half) is absorbed. If they take a larger dose, say twelve grams orally, only about two grams is absorbed if the individual is healthy. A cat, which has a low rate of synthesis compared to some animals, makes the equivalent of two and a half grams, comparable to an oral dose of twelve grams or more in a human.

The high dose hypothesis, which proposes that ascorbate is required in doses substantially higher than needed to prevent scurvy, is as valid as the low dose hypothesis described in the previous section.

Evidence for the high dose hypothesis might include:

- Showing that a deficiency disease exists at lower doses

- Showing that measures of "good health" are maximal with high intakes

- Showing that lower doses are toxic or in some way deleterious

- Showing that animals with high intakes are more resistant to stress

- Showing that animals with high intakes are more resistant to infection

- Showing that animals with high intakes are more resistant to degenerative disease

- Showing that animals synthesise ascorbate in large amounts

- As ascorbate is an antioxidant, showing that high doses produce a more favourable redox balance

- Demonstrating that competing low dose hypotheses are invalid.

Other factors may be included in this list. Unlike those for the low dose hypothesis, some of the factors have substantial supporting evidence, for example, the lack of toxicity. Once again, the most powerful feature in this list is to refute the competing low dose hypotheses. Refutation is more powerful than supporting evidence. The most convincing evidence for high doses would be to show that low doses are unhelpful, deleterious or lead to deficiency disease. A person promoting high, gram level doses needs to show that lower doses are suboptimal.

# Dynamic flow

The dynamic flow model offers an alternative to the low dose and high dose hypotheses. It is a modification of the high dose ideas of Irwin Stone and Linus Pauling. It also incorporates Dr Robert Cathcart's ideas and suggestions for the mechanism of action of high-dose ascorbate. The dynamic flow model depends upon the two-phase pharmacokinetic characteristics of ascorbate in plasma.

## Two-phase pharmacokinetics

At low concentrations of ascorbate in the blood plasma, below about 70 microM/L, the kidneys reabsorb vitamin C from the urine.[38,15,17] At higher levels, the kidneys allow ascorbate to "overflow" into urine, and more is lost. This is what we mean by two-phase pharmacokinetics – a slow loss phase, at low concentrations, and a faster loss phase, when the concentration is higher. Both the NIH and the RDA committees have ignored these dual phases in their reports of ascorbate blood plasma concentrations.

Transporters in the kidney reabsorb ascorbate when plasma levels are low. The RDA committee has indicated that little ascorbate is excreted with doses up to 80mg per day. Some breakdown products of ascorbate are excreted at this intake. The committee states that the biological half-life varies, from 8-40 days, and is inversely related to the body pool.[8] This figure is correct, though incomplete and selective. It applies only to the low-concentration (slow loss) phase in plasma. The reason for this long half-life is the active re-absorption of ascorbate by the kidneys, which helps the body avoid acute scurvy by not excreting ascorbate when it is in short supply.

If ascorbate is abundant, the half-life is very short. Above a plasma baseline level of about 70 microM/L, the kidney transporters are saturated and ascorbate is excreted rapidly. Based on the NIH experiments, the half-life of ascorbate is about 30 minutes. Following a large injected dose, half the dose is excreted within half an hour.

The RDA committee uses this rapid excretion of ascorbate, incorrectly, as a primary criterion for limiting intake. Both the NIH and the RDA committee failed to appreciate the two-phase nature of the concentration of ascorbate in blood plasma. Blood is the main supply route for ascorbate in the body. Ultimately, tissues receive ascorbate that is absorbed from the blood plasma. The blood plasma's response to changing ascorbate levels is therefore a central feature in understanding the body's requirements. The NIH, who included plasma steady state "saturation" in their studies, recognise this fact.[15,32] However, the RDA committee based its recommendation on neutrophil "saturation", a more static measure.[o]

## Equivalence of higher doses

In healthy adults, all doses above about 500mg produce similar plasma concentration curves. Little is gained by increasing a single dose from 500mg to, say, 2000mg, as the amount absorbed and blood levels are similar. In this respect, it could be claimed that doses above 500mg are essentially wasted. However, this is not true if the subject has even a minor stress or illness, as more of the larger dose is then absorbed. The RDA committee provided no evidence that they understood how ascorbate absorption varies with the person's state of health.

## Bowel tolerance

The dynamic flow model incorporates Cathcart's principle of bowel tolerance.[49] The RDA committee did not address this point. The bowel tolerance is the dose of vitamin C that causes diarrhoea. Bowel tolerance and, by direct implication, the amount of a dose absorbed, increase dramatically during illness and stress. The RDA committee suggests that unabsorbed ascorbate in the gut causes diarrhoea. Thus, if diarrhoea is absent, the high dose has been absorbed. This increase in absorption can vary from about two grams to 200 grams. In any population, there will be stressed or sick people and the bowel tolerance will differ greatly from one individual to another.

---

o It could be that the committee members realised they could recommend lower intakes if this measure was taken to be the primary criterion.

# Return to mammalian physiology

Dynamic flow restores human physiology to the condition of animals that synthesise their own vitamin C.[9] Since people are unable to synthesise vitamin C, they cannot make more when requirements increase. When stressed, people use more ascorbate. It can take many grams per day, over a period of weeks, to restore plasma levels. This is consistent with observations on the bowel tolerance, which indicate greater need. The plasma measurements by the NIH and others, cited by the RDA committee, relate to normal, healthy, young adults and may grossly underestimate requirements for many people.

The dynamic flow model suggests that people need to ingest vitamin C frequently enough to maintain a constant, dynamic flow through the body. According to this model, the human body requires an over-supply of vitamin C, to act as a reservoir in times of increased need. The low dose hypothesis and RDA model view excretion as wasteful, but do not explain why animals that make their own vitamin C in large amounts also excrete it, rather than just making less. At first sight, this excretion might seem inefficient: the sick animal uses energy to make extra ascorbate and then loses it in urine. An alternative interpretation is the higher levels of ascorbate, and its loss, provide a valuable physiological function that assists in overcoming stress. An analogy would be increased temperature or fever, which uses energy but can help overcome bacterial infection. In the dynamic flow model, excretion is a sign that the inbuilt redundancy of the system is ready to compensate for any sudden deficit. The amount needed varies according to the individual's genetic constitution, nutritional status, level of stress, state of health or illness, and so on.

The dynamic flow model provides a consistent margin of safety against disease.[9] In dynamic flow, there is unabsorbed ascorbate in the gut. Some ascorbate enters the bloodstream, flows through the body and is excreted in the urine.[P] The intake should be such that the plasma is normally in a steady state

---

[P] The flow of ascorbate carries antioxidant electrons, which are available to prevent oxidation and keep other free radical scavengers in a reduced state.

condition, at a level above the 70 microM/L baseline for prevention of acute scurvy. When stress occurs, the requirement is increased and more is absorbed from the reservoir in the gut. The increased absorption takes the place of the synthesis that occurs in other mammals.

## Pharmacokinetics and dose levels

A large oral dose of ascorbate is only partly absorbed from the gut. To achieve dynamic flow, each dose should exceed about 200mg to ensure raised plasma levels. A single dose will increase blood plasma levels, reaching a peak after about 2-3 hours. After this, blood plasma levels fall back to baseline values. The short half-life of higher doses of ascorbate means that oral doses are eliminated within a few hours.

Dynamic flow requires the plasma ascorbate concentration to reach a steady state, above the depletion baseline. Repeated doses of ascorbate, taken at intervals of similar size, result in a steady state. A pharmacological heuristic for achieving steady state levels is that the dose interval should not be greater than five half-lives. For ascorbate, this means oral doses about every three hours. If this is not practical, then the use of sustained release formulations might allow the interval between doses to be extended.

According to the NIH data, the maximum steady state concentration of ascorbate in blood plasma is above 220 microM/L.[50] The NIH paper indicates that this steady state concentration can be achieved by taking three grams every four hours. Previous studies by the NIH stated that blood plasma was "saturated" at about 70 microM/L.[15,17] However, in view of the higher concentrations described in their later studies,[50] this was clearly incorrect. The maximum steady state concentration achievable with oral doses in a healthy young adult could typically be higher than the NIH figure, in the region of 250 microM/L.[38,50,46]

Given that all single doses above 500mg lead to similar plasma concentrations for an adult in good health, we can estimate that a minimum dose of 500mg, every four hours, would provide a quasi steady state. This would be reasonably close to the maximum value, perhaps around 200 microM/L. In other words, a dose of three grams per day, taken as six equally spaced half-gram doses, could result in blood levels similar to the steady state values obtained by the NIH. This would be a minimum dose to provide a pseudo steady state plasma level, varying slightly and somewhat short of "saturation".[Q] It may be that higher or more frequent doses would provide additional benefit at the onset of illness, but here we are looking for the lowest dose consistent with the NIH concept of plasma saturation.

## Implications

The dynamic flow hypothesis has profound implications for the ascorbate intake debate. Firstly, most scientific studies have used single daily supplements. These would raise the blood plasma levels, and thus be effective, for only a small fraction of the day. Studies that claimed no effect on, say, the common cold may have grossly underestimated the true potential. A person could catch a cold and the infection could take hold while their blood levels were low. Most conductors of clinical studies have ignored the short half-life of ascorbate; the results of these studies are biased and misleading. We predict that studies using the dynamic flow protocol will show greater benefits than those using once or twice daily doses.

## Explanation of high dose effects

Some experiments on high dose vitamin C have failed to show a positive effect on immune function. We could predict this variability, as many studies used a single daily dose and ignored the short half-life of ascorbate in the blood. However, since the committee believed the half-life of vitamin C was greater than eight days, they suggested that the lack of effect was because the subject's white blood cells were already saturated at a low dose (100mg per day), so higher doses provided no additional benefit. We will show that this explanation is mistaken. Paradoxically, the committee accepts that many high-dose studies show large effects. Every. positive result refutes the hypothesis that doses above 100mg per day are worthless.

---

[Q] To achieve steady-state plasma values, the dose interval should really be less than 2.5 hours.

The dynamic flow model offers a consistent explanation of the variation in experimental results. Because of the short half-life, single high doses only increase plasma levels for a small fraction of the day. Given this short half-life, the positive results are surprising, as the dosing regimen is not consistent with maximum effectiveness. Since some positive results are found, even with infrequent doses, we predict that frequent doses, in line with the dynamic flow model, would be even more valuable.

# Saturation

The RDA committee base their vitamin C recommendations largely on what they refer to as "saturation". Many people have misunderstood the nature of this term: they think it means that the body cannot absorb more vitamin C than is specified by the RDA. The use of the term saturation is misleading. Here we cover the possible meanings of the word saturation, in relationship to vitamin C intake.

Firstly, we should be aware that the use of vitamin C "saturation" as a criterion for setting the RDA is an assumption, and is not justified by the evidence. Presumably, the committee assume that the body is a static system in which the requirement for vitamin C is unchanging. If this were true, then if the healthy body were saturated, that would be enough. However, it is not true: under conditions of stress, shock or illness, the body can exhaust its available ascorbate rapidly and require gram-level doses for weeks before blood levels are restored.[9]

## Chemical saturation

When the word saturation occurs in a scientific context, the most obvious assumption is that we are talking about chemical saturation. According to the rules of chemistry, a saturated solution contains all of the substance that it is capable of dissolving; it is a solution of a substance in equilibrium with an excess of undissolved substance. Vitamin C is highly soluble in water. The human body, which contains a high proportion of water, does not reach anything close to chemical saturation with the consumption of a few hundred milligrams of vitamin C per day. A person could not consume enough vitamin C to make their body chemically saturated.

## Enzyme saturation

In biology, the word saturation is used in relation to enzymes. Enzymes are protein molecules that speed up, or catalyse, a chemical reaction.[51] The centre of action of an enzyme is its receptor, a section of the molecule (the active site) shaped like the substance on which it acts (the substrate). This fitting together of the enzyme and the substrate makes biochemical reactions very specific. The usual analogy is that if the molecule is like a key, the enzyme is the lock into which it fits. When the lock and key are joined, the enzyme enables a reaction and the molecule is released in its changed form. A chemical reaction has occurred.

The action of enzymes depends on the attachment and release of the substrate. If there is a lot of substrate relative to the amount of enzyme, all the active sites can be occupied by substrate molecules. The enzyme is then said to be saturated with substrate, and the rate of reaction is a maximum.

While vitamin C is involved in many enzymatic reactions in the body, this is not the form of saturation used for justifying the RDA.

## Ascorbate transporter saturation

Many cells have biochemical pumps on their surfaces, to transport ascorbate or its oxidised form, dehydroascorbate.[52] The molecular configuration of dehydroascorbate is similar to that of the sugar glucose, so glucose transporters (GLUT) can convey it. Ascorbate specific transporters (SVCT)[R] also exist in some cells. These transporters have similar characteristics to enzymes; they increase the rate of movement of the molecules across the cell membrane. Transporter proteins are subject to substrate saturation, in a similar way to standard enzymes. The type of transporters, the number of pumps in the cell membrane and the rate of transport determine the concentration of ascorbate within a number of cell types. Ascorbate may also enter cells by other means, such as diffusion, and such mechanisms may be dominant in some cells.

The plasma baseline level corresponds to the saturation of kidney transporters, which reabsorb ascorbate up to this level. Saturation of white blood cells, and some other cell types, depends on transporters in the outer cell membrane. Therefore, the saturation of neutrophils, which the RDA committee claim is

---

[R] Sodium dependent Vitamin C Transporter

the justification for the RDA, is indirectly related to transporter saturation.

## Drug receptor saturation

Many drugs act on receptors in a highly specific way. A drug is shaped like its receptor, in the same way that an enzyme is shaped like its substrate. Drug receptors become saturated in the presence of large amounts of drug, just as the active site of an enzyme becomes saturated with its substrate. High levels of ascorbate, which are used to treat disease, could be considered as a drug or pharmacologically active substance. However, the principal function of ascorbate is as an electron donor or antioxidant, and this does not normally involve drug receptors. This form of saturation is therefore not relevant to the justification of the RDA.

## Household or physical saturation

One form of saturation with which we are all familiar is that of the simple household sponge. A sponge will absorb water up to a finite limit, at which point it is described as saturated. This simple physical form of saturation does not have the characteristics of the saturation used in the RDA justification.

## Physiological saturation

Physiological saturation is a form of holistic pseudo-saturation that is more difficult to define. According to Mark Levine, of the NIH, plasma saturation refers to "the sum of the biological processes of bioavailability, tissue transport, and renal excretion".[53] This form of saturation depends on the physiological and biochemical factors that, together, limit the maximum concentration of a substance in the body, tissues or cells. As far as we can tell, in their justification document the RDA committee refer to physiological saturation, which is difficult to define in a clear and unambiguous way.

Even given the weakness of these criteria, the body is not saturated at a dose of 200mg per day.[9] Physiological saturation should equate to maximum steady state levels. Otherwise, the term saturation is meaningless.

We can subdivide physiological saturation into different categories:

- **Body saturation**: pseudo-saturation of the human body taken as a whole

- **Tissue saturation**: pseudo-saturation of an organ of the body or a particular tissue

- **Cell saturation**: pseudo-saturation of a particular cell type, for example red blood cells

- **Plasma saturation**: pseudo-saturation of the fluid within a compartment of the body, for example blood plasma.

The RDA committee has selected body saturation as their preferred measure. This is a static concept, which may not be adequate as a measure of physiological need. For example, it does not take account of the increased requirements in people who are ill or stressed. Moreover, body saturation is difficult to estimate, so the committee elected not to use a direct measurement. Instead, they used saturation of a particular cell type, neutrophil white blood cells, as an estimator of general tissue saturation, which they then extrapolated implicitly to the whole body.

## Concept manipulation

The RDA committee provide no valid biological reasons for their choice of saturation as an indicator for human requirements. In particular, they use a single, fixed value for saturation, whereas requirements may vary rapidly. We note that the nature of the term saturation implies a limiting measure and thus provides a "marketing strategy" for restricting consideration of higher intakes.

# Plasma vitamin C concentrations

Blood plasma vitamin C concentrations provide an indication of ascorbate requirements. Unlike white blood cell saturation, plasma ascorbate levels reflect the rapidly changing intake and requirements of the body.

## Steady state plasma concentrations

Experiments by Dr Mark Levine's research group at the NIH form the primary data included in the RDA justification. The RDA committee commended these plasma measurements as unique, for their use of

> "rigorous criteria for achieving steady state plasma concentrations".

However, these experiments were flawed, in both design and interpretation.

To start with, the NIH pharmacokinetic study had *no control subjects or measures.* The RDA committee failed to notice this lack, although they reject studies with inadequate controls when those studies show positive effects for high doses of ascorbate. Their position might have been stronger had they noticed that the central basis of their recommendations, the NIH studies, also had no controls.

The first NIH study measured plasma and white blood cell levels in seven (7) healthy, young adults.[15] This number of subjects is too small for reliable statistical analysis or to act as a representative sample for the population as a whole. Scientifically, the paper is equivalent to a short series of observational case studies. Perhaps the fact that it contains repeated measurements, with estimates of statistical variation, confused the RDA committee into thinking it was a substantial piece of work. However, this simple observational study used an inadequate sample, invalid experimental methods and a misleading analysis of the data.[9]

The NIH followed their pharmacokinetic study on seven males with a study of 15 young, adult females.[17] This was also an uncontrolled, observational study, with the same methodological errors.

## Poor experimental design

The NIH experiments purport to show that plasma becomes saturated with a vitamin C intake of 1000mg or less.[15,17] To show this, the researchers gave a dose of vitamin C and waited 12 hours, before measuring the plasma levels. Using this procedure, they found that increasing the dose did not greatly increase blood levels; instead, the levels reached what the NIH called a "steady state". Rather than realising this was because the subject had already excreted the dose, the NIH claimed it was because the body was saturated, so higher doses were redundant. This is a ridiculous error, for a group of scientists whose own data demonstrate the short half-life of ascorbate. Unfortunately, the NIH study was highly influential within the medical establishment, before we revealed its flaws, eight years later.[9]

The following diagram, taken from the book *Ascorbate*,[9] shows the difference between what Levine's NIH group called a "steady state", and a true pharmacological steady state.

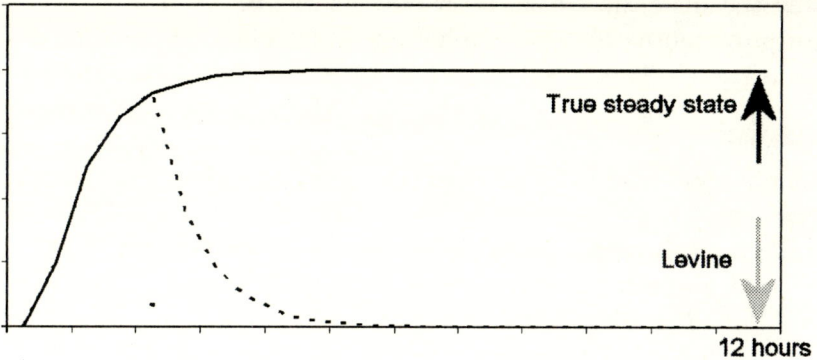

**True steady state**

**Levine**

**12 hours**

This schematic graph was computed from vitamin C absorption and excretion data.[54] It shows levels of ascorbate above base level (~70 microM/L) and illustrates the NIH's "steady state" error. Numerical plasma concentrations were omitted to illustrate that the shape of these curves is consistent over a large range of doses.

- - - The dotted line shows a single two-gram dose taken at time zero, and the grey arrow shows what Levine measured.

—— The solid line shows a two-gram dose followed by repeated dosing (one gram per hour). A steady state (of about 240-250 microM/L) is reached within a few hours with these doses. Notice how the steady state value is higher than the maximum value for a single dose. The darker arrow shows a true steady state measurement.

A large oral dose of vitamin C increases plasma concentrations to a maximum in two to three hours, after which the blood levels drop.[9] The NIH researchers measured minimum or background levels, but claimed they were measuring "saturated" (or maximum) levels. Mistaking the minimum for the maximum produces the largest error possible with these measurements.

The NIH claimed to have measured steady state saturation of plasma, which did not increase with the oral dose. As we have seen, what they actually measured was the background level, after most of the dose had been excreted. In pharmacology, a steady state refers to a constant blood concentration, which does not change with time. The NIH did not demonstrate a steady state, but a waveform, repeated every 12 hours. The levels rose after the dose, declining as it was excreted. They measured the minimum point on this waveform, then claimed it represented "saturation". The blood was not saturated: even graphs in the same paper show higher levels that those given this misnomer. However, both the NIH and the RDA committees failed to notice this obvious discrepancy. The RDA committee indicated a steady state had been achieved, thus endorsing the NIH's errors. Unfortunately, many people thought the NIH had shown that low doses of ascorbate saturate the blood (i.e. chemical saturation). This misunderstanding became widespread, leading to the belief that high doses of vitamin C are a waste of money.

The NIH performed further studies on plasma levels, in which the researchers considered repeated ascorbate doses, three grams every four hours.[55] They reported a steady state of 220 microM, which is three times the concentration they previously claimed as "saturated". Once again, they did not notice the discrepancy. The NIH has not retracted its claim that plasma is saturated at 70 microM/L, even though these errors have been pointed out to them. Instead, they redefine the word "saturated" to mean something quite different from what most scientists would expect it to mean. By doing this, they spread confusion among scientists and the public alike.

Based on the NIH's own data, it would take 18 grams per day, in divided doses, for blood plasma to reach a physiological, pseudo-saturated steady state.[55] Such a dose should give a plasma level of 220 microM/L. Therefore, using the NIH criterion of plasma saturation, together with their own data (analysed correctly), we arrive at an RDA in the region of 20 grams per day, in divided doses. This value is more than 200 times the current RDA.

The RDA committee has accepted the NIH results at face value. Since the RDA committee were taken in by such obvious errors, we are forced to question their scientific judgement. Now we have provided a reinterpretation of the NIH data, the RDA committee should be required to explain why their RDA recommendation is only 0.5% of the intake required to achieve a genuine (steady state) physiological saturation of plasma.

# Bioavailability

When people hear the term bioavailability, they are likely to think it means the amount of vitamin C that is available to the tissues or, even, the amount that the cells can actually use. The implication is that reduced bioavailability limits the usefulness of ascorbate. Several people have described their understanding to us in these terms. These included scientists and physicians, who should have known better. Despite the name, it is not a measure of biological availability or usefulness: *bioavailability is the proportion of an oral dose that is absorbed from the gut.*

The concept of "bioavailability" is misleading when applied to ascorbate. The term is an estimate of the proportion of an oral dose that is absorbed. If a person takes a low dose of ascorbate (30-180mg), about 80% of the dose is absorbed (24-144mg).[34,35,56] If they take a single higher dose (one gram), then the body absorbs a lower proportion (50%), even though the absolute amount absorbed is greater (500mg).[7,15,32,57] The RDA committee have only a small section on bioavailability in their justification document, but appear to have misunderstood its implications. This may have biased the rest of their study against higher doses.

Bioavailability measures absorption from the gut. The RDA committee suggest that this absorption occurs in the intestines by means of active transport. This may not be the only route, or even the dominant one. Vitamin C is a weak, organic acid, and such acids are normally absorbed rapidly through the stomach.[58] The committee do not explain why they believe that specific transporters lower in the gut dominate the absorption of ascorbate, or how this relates to the rapid absorption which has been observed.

Bioavailability is the relative amount in the plasma obtained from an oral dose, compared to an equal dose administered by intravenous injection:

**Bioavailability =** <u>**Plasma level from oral dose**</u> **x 100%**
**Plasma level from injected dose**

For example, suppose that by taking a one gram dose orally, the plasma vitamin C was only half that gained from a one gram intravenous dose. The bioavailability of the oral dose would be 50%. Only half of the oral dose has reached the blood, the rest has not been absorbed.

To see how the concept of bioavailability is biased against higher doses, suppose the absolute plasma level with a 500mg oral dose was the same as that for a 1000mg dose. The bioavailability for the 1000mg dose would only be half that of the 500mg dose, because the injected dose would be twice as large for the larger dose. In this example, the blood levels are identical, but the bioavailability of the smaller dose is twice that of the larger.

Despite the impressive name, bioavailability is at best a reflection of the absorption of oral doses of vitamin C. Furthermore, the bioavailability of a given dose is not a fixed attribute: it can vary. Since the amount of vitamin C absorbed depends on the person's state of health, there is variation both between individuals and within the same individual. Thus, the idea that a certain dose of ascorbate has a fixed bioavailability is faulty. The bioavailability of large doses, in particular, increases if a person is ill or stressed.

Large doses of vitamin C have a short half-life, about 30 minutes. Bioavailability is also transient, because no sooner has the vitamin C been absorbed, than it starts to be excreted. For this reason, it does not make sense to apply the idea of bioavailability to daily doses. Consider some examples, starting with the case of dividing a daily dose in two. Two separate doses, taken a few hours apart within a single day, act independently because of the short half-life of ascorbate. Now, suppose bioavailability was 100% at 200mg. If someone took two 200mg doses, 12 hours apart, these would be independent, so each would have a bioavailability of 100%. Therefore, this divided 400mg dose also has a bioavailability of 100%, whereas a single 400mg dose has a lower bioavailability. Four doses six hours apart would also be relatively independent, as the majority of the previous dose would have been excreted by the time the next was taken. Thus, a daily intake of 800mg could have a bioavailability approaching 100%, if taken in divided doses.[S]

Dividing a daily dose into several smaller doses increases its bioavailability dramatically. The RDA committee did not refer to the dosing schedule when they discussed absorption. By not indicating or appreciating the importance of the short half-life of high-dose vitamin C, the committee misrepresented the basic absorptive mechanism for oral doses.

The RDA committee did not appear to realise that bioavailability could not be considered without addressing Cathcart's well-known principle of bowel tolerance limits.[49] This shows that absorption of ascorbate varies within a single individual, increasing dramatically during stress.[59] The RDA committee suggest that the diarrhoea produced by large doses is caused by the osmotic action of the unabsorbed ascorbate in the gut. They would thus presumably agree that if the diarrhoea is absent, then the high dose has been absorbed. This increase in absorption, and hence "bioavailability", can be as great as two orders of magnitude. In any population, there will be stressed or sick people. The committee's failure to cover the topic of bowel tolerance suggests their selection of data on absorption was biased.

The NIH measured "bioavailability" and suggested it was complete at a dose of 200mg.[15,17] The RDA committee considered "bioavailability" as a factor affecting the vitamin C requirement. Their report did not indicate any of the limitations of this measurement and used it, incorrectly, as a support for low doses.

## Increased bowel tolerance

The well-established phenomenon of increased bowel tolerance with stress or illness is one of the most interesting observations about vitamin C. Cathcart's description of increased bowel tolerance has been confirmed many times. We can postulate that the increased absorption of vitamin C is a mechanism that has evolved to assist recovery from illness in

---

[S] There would be a little overlap between the plasma responses for these doses, which lowers the estimated bioavailability.

animals that cannot synthesise ascorbate. These mechanisms have yet to be investigated fully.

A type of glucose transporter, GLUT4, which also pumps dehydroascorbate, responds to insulin. Normally a large proportion of GLUT4 pumps are contained within the cell body. The hormone insulin, which signals high external glucose, triggers movement of GLUT4 transporters from the cell body to the outer cell membrane. When they reach the outer membrane, the GLUT4 can pump glucose (and dehydroascorbate) into the cell. Insulin thus acts as a signal to increase the uptake of glucose and dehydroascorbate. This mechanism may provide a model for increased bowel ascorbate tolerance during illness. Insulin and some other hormones increase during stressful conditions, and may trigger the transport of ascorbate into the body. This transport is unlikely to be by way of GLUT4 pumps, as it has not been reported that these are present and performing this function in the gut. However, the presence of a hormone-sensitive ascorbate transporter would explain the increased uptake phenomenon.

# Excretion

The RDA committee consider excretion to be a central factor in determining human requirements. Before we discuss excretion of ascorbate, consider the case of water. Unless dehydrated, a person who drinks a large glass of water will excrete an equivalent amount. However, this does not mean that a subject who is not thirsty or dehydrated does not need water. Nor does it mean that water has no physiological function, since it is excreted. Doctors advise us to drink about 1.5-2 litres of water a day, for good health. If we decided to adjust our intake of water to a level that would prevent loss through excretion, we would find ourselves in danger of kidney damage. The dynamic flow of water through the body is a physiological requirement.

The RDA committee do not discuss the biological implications of the finding that the kidney excretes high plasma levels of ascorbate. The committee's assumption appears to be that excreted ascorbate is, and has been, of no use to the body. Presumably, they consider this obvious, as in the old "expensive urine" jibe, used against high-dose supplementation. This is an unwarranted assumption. Excretion is a central feature of both the dynamic flow model and Cathcart's proposed mechanism for the action of ascorbate in disease.[59]

The majority of other mammals, which synthesise ascorbate in their tissues, make large amounts, equivalent to many grams in humans. This synthesis is internal, so their ascorbate does not have to be absorbed through the gut. The amount synthesised is equivalent to an intravenous dose of several grams in humans. Oral doses are not absorbed well in the healthy, so it would be harder to achieve the same levels with supplementation. Mammals have in their kidneys similar transporters to those in humans; like humans, these animals also excrete ascorbate.[60,61] Moreover, this excretion increases during illness.[9] The re-absorption of vitamin C by the kidney uses SVCT transporters, specific to the reduced form of ascorbate.[62] This means that the oxidised form of vitamin C, dehydroascorbate, is preferentially lost. This is a central feature of the dynamic flow theory, in which good health relies on maintaining the ratio of ascorbate to dehydroascorbate at a high level.

Unwisely, the RDA committee used urinary excretion as a primary consideration for the RDA. They did not explain why human physiology should differ from that of other mammals. They did not explain why animals manufacture, and then excrete, ascorbate, apparently wasting precious resources and energy. In addition, they did not explain the observation that this apparently wasteful process increases, along with ascorbate synthesis, when the animal is ill. They provided no evidence that the excretion of ascorbate in humans is not a beneficial part of normal physiology, honed by millions of years of evolution, as in other mammals.

# Toxicity

Vitamin C is classified as "generally regarded as safe" (GRAS). This means that the US Food and Drugs Administration recognise the safety of ascorbate.[63] Its toxicity is low.[T] We can compare the toxicity of ascorbate to that of water.[9] Both are essential to the human body and we would die if we did not have enough. However, it would probably be easier to kill yourself by overdosing on water than oral ascorbate. While reports of deaths from drinking too much water are rare, they do occur. However, we could not find a single reported death from ingesting too much ascorbate.

High doses of ascorbate are remarkably non-toxic. In their report, the RDA committee reject suggestions that high levels of ascorbate cause the following problems:

- Kidney stone formation

- Excess iron formation

- Reduced vitamin B12 and copper levels

- Increased oxygen demand

- Systemic conditioning (rebound scurvy)

- Pro-oxidant effects

- Dental enamel erosion

- Allergic response

These conclusions are similar to those of Levine at the NIH.[64] Levine suggests a theoretical possibility that increased urinary oxalate could lead to a low incidence of kidney stones in a large population, although the evidence appears slight.[15,17]

---

[T] Sigma-Aldrich, a leading supplier of chemicals for life science laboratories, lists the oral LD50 for ascorbate in the rat as 11,900mg/kg, which scales to 1.2kg in a 100kg human. (For comparison, the oral LD50 for common salt in the rat is only 3,000mg/kg.)

Millions of people have been self-supplementing with gram level doses for years, with an excellent safety record.

It is possible that rare subgroups, people with conditions such as kidney disease, haemochromatosis or glucose-6-phosphatase deficiency, could be more susceptible to toxic effects. However, this has not been established. The appropriate dose in such cases may be more a medical matter than a nutritional consideration. Physicians should guide the nutrition of patients with kidney disease, for example.

The possibility of toxicity is a serious factor for any RDA recommendation. In the case of ascorbate, the only reliable toxic effects mentioned by the RDA committees are mild gastrointestinal upsets and diarrhoea, following large doses. Gastric irritation can be ameliorated by taking mineral formulations, such as sodium ascorbate, rather than ascorbic acid. A high concentration of vitamin C draws water into the gut through osmosis, which causes the stools to become loose. Both low- and high-dose proponents agree that this occurs, but differ in their interpretation. The RDA committee takes these effects as indications of a toxic limit to intake. By contrast, Dr Robert Cathcart uses the bowel tolerance level as an indicator of the subject's state of health. High doses of vitamin C provide a safe alternative to drug based laxatives, dietary fibre or prunes: arguably, this is a side-benefit rather than a toxic effect.

## Tolerable upper limit

The tolerable upper limit is the highest level of daily nutrient that is likely to pose no risk of adverse effects in almost all individuals. The absolute nature of the notion of "no risk" hardly belongs in biology. Rather, the risk should be considered in terms of an estimated low or negligible probability.

The RDA committee have set their upper limit at two grams per day, based on mild gastrointestinal upset. In the absence of tangible data on side effects, they based their limit on causation of loose stools. The committee accept that this minor side effect is not serious, is self-limiting, and is soon eased if the dose is reduced. There are no other established side effects of high doses.

The committee estimated that the limit (Lowest Observed Adverse Effect Level) for loose stools in an adult would occur with doses of about three grams. They did not specify the method or frequency of dosage. This is important, because although a person might get diarrhoea from a single three gram dose, if they took the same dose, split into several portions and spread throughout the day, they would be less likely to feel any gastrointestinal discomfort. The committee then estimated a lower value (No Observed Adverse Effect Level), which they placed at two grams. They did not explain the origins of this estimate; it was derived using an "uncertainty" or "fudge" factor. The uncertainty factor was 1.5, suggesting they chose it to give an answer in round numbers.[U]

The committee chose diarrhoea as their criterion for the upper limit. However, this effect varies greatly between different people. For a few healthy people it might be three grams, as suggested by the committee. For some people, it may be as high as 30 grams, depending on the dosing schedule. Furthermore, the moment a person gets ill, the level increases dramatically. Therefore, it makes biological sense to set the upper limit separately for each individual.

People can determine their own upper limit; it is the same as Cathcart's bowel tolerance level.[49] Thus, if we take individual variation into account, the difference between the RDA committee's tolerable upper limits and the highest levels suggested for megadose supplementation can be reconciled. By this argument, if we accept that there will be "no observed adverse effect" at two grams per day, the upper limit for healthy people (determined on an individual basis) will be in the range of two to 20 grams per day. This suggestion is consistent with the European Union recommendations; the EU Scientific Committee for Food (1993) indicated a maximum intake in a similar range, one to 10 grams each day.[2] It is also consistent with the proposals for high dose supplementation.[9,10,38]

The committee's justification for their "tolerable upper limit" essentially endorses Cathcart's approach to supplementation. The committee probably did not realise that their method for determination of the tolerable upper limit

---

[U] The calculation was 3/1.5 = 2 grams.

suggests such high doses, when individual variation is taken into account.

## Risk

The committee indicate that the probability of adverse effects from vitamin C supplements in the gram range appears to be very low. However, they also indicate that people should not be advised to exceed the tolerable upper limit routinely; they give no reason for this suggestion. We can agree with this suggestion, but only if people determine their own individual bowel tolerance limit and are aware that it can change. If a person feels unwell or has a cold coming on, then the bowel tolerance limit will increase. In these circumstances, people can determine their current bowel tolerance using Cathcart's method.

## Conclusions

The existence of a tolerable upper limit could deter research into higher vitamin C doses. The RDA committee suggest that intake above the upper limit may be appropriate for investigation within well-controlled clinical trials, adding that, in the light of evaluating possible benefits to health, clinical trials of doses above the upper limit should not be discouraged. However, we shall see later that the committee have themselves discouraged such trials in cancer and heart disease, by suggesting that subjects should be pre-screened to have intakes of less than 90mg per day.

The toxicity of ascorbate is a critical factor for determining optimal intake, as the possible benefits are balanced against the potential for harm. Most experts agree that ascorbate is one of the safest substances known. There could be a low possibility of harmful effects such as kidney stones from extremely high doses in a few sensitive individuals, which is a factor to weigh against potential benefits. However, the level of safety is such that even a relatively low probability of benefit would dominate a cost-benefit analysis.

The committee members have, in effect, used Cathcart's bowel tolerance technique to determine the tolerable upper limit. If they applied this procedure individually, rather than estimating one figure for the entire population, the new upper limits would be consistent with the highest doses suggested by advocates of vitamin C supplementation.

# Measures of oxidation

The primary role of ascorbate in the body is as a donor of electrons. It acts as an antioxidant. Doses of vitamin C of one gram and above provide increased antioxidant protection in plasma.[65] Each molecule of ascorbate can donate two electrons, to reduce an oxidising free radical.

There are many possible measures of oxidation damage in the body.[66] The concentration of ascorbate[67] or the ratio to its oxidised form, dehydroascorbate, provides a measure of the redox state of a tissue. Similarly, the ratio of the antioxidant glutathione to its oxidised form is another measure of oxidative stress.[68] As ascorbate prevents such oxidation, these ratios might be used to indicate a minimum intake, but the committee did not report consideration of this option.

The RDA committee agrees that ascorbate can reduce most physiologically relevant free radicals.[69] They suggest that neutrophils are 80 percent saturated at an intake of 75mg, adding that this should protect them from oxidative injury when activated during infections and inflammation.[70,71] Their own description of the use of ascorbate during white blood cell activation (described later) indicates that this statement is incorrect, as the cells require high plasma levels to function optimally.

Notably, the oxidation of white blood cells is given a separate section in the US RDA report.[8] This is consistent with these cells having unusual and specific ascorbate requirements, with specialised absorption and biochemistry.

# Immune function

The RDA committee came to ridiculous conclusions with respect to ascorbate and immune function. There is a widespread scientific debate concerning the utility of ascorbate in prevention and treatment of infectious disease.[9,11] This debate has been side-stepped by the committee, who avoided it by examining only selected (mainly low-dose) data.

The committee admits that doses of ascorbate, in the range 200mg to six grams a day, influence the immune response in humans. Such doses enhance the actions of anti-microbial and killer cells, promote the proliferation of lymphocytes, stimulate chemotaxis, and delay dermal sensitivity. The dose range mentioned is well above the RDA. There appears to be little dispute that ascorbate at high doses can strengthen the immune response.

The committee points out that there have been few controlled studies on the action of ascorbate on infections in humans. At first sight, this statement might appear conservative. However, despite numerous reports of the efficacy of high-dose vitamins over half a century, the medical establishment has avoided performing clinical trials or funding the experiments of others. Observations on the positive response to vitamin C of patients with severe infections are common in the literature.[9,10,31,61,48] These observations are by multiple, independent investigators, including Drs Kalokerinos and Brighthope in Australia, and Drs Cathcart and Riordan in the US. The magnitude of the response is substantial and is not easily explained by placebo effect or investigator bias. Reports and studies of the efficacy of high-dose ascorbate have been reviewed recently in Dr Tom Levy's book.[11] Levy's book is a description of the reported action of vitamin C in a host of disease processes. The reports are often astounding, and include recovery from AIDS and cures of metastatic cancer.[v]

By selective examination of the data, the committee concluded that the evidence that supplemental vitamin C has a significant effect on immune function is not convincing.

---

[v] In physics and other areas of science, repeated independent observations of this magnitude would be considered indicators for urgent research.

# White blood cells

Ascorbate levels in white blood cells form the core of the RDA justification. The RDA committee accepts that white blood cells, along with the adrenals, pituitary and the lens of the eye, contain the highest measured ascorbate levels in the body. The committee claims that white blood cell levels reflect levels in the body pool and the liver. However, the evidence for this claim comes from other species (monkeys and guinea pigs), rather than human studies. In addition, the single paper cited for this claim is tentative.[39]

## Body pool

If people are in good health, the total amount of vitamin C in their bodies is relatively static. Intermittent high-level supplementation does not increase the body pool greatly, although this may not be the case with the more sustained plasma levels achieved in dynamic flow. Tissues that absorb ascorbate actively, using transporters (pumps) in their cell membranes, dominate the body pool. The tissues with the highest ascorbate concentrations are specialised in relation to their ascorbate biochemistry.[38] They contain large numbers of transporters, which concentrate and retain ascorbate. Even when levels in the local environment are low, the transporters pump ascorbate into the cells, against the concentration gradient.

Transporters in the kidneys re-absorb ascorbate when it falls below a minimum level, stopping it from being lost in the urine. Kidney re-absorption provides the body's first line of defence against scurvy. Similarly, the tissues that are most sensitive to depletion have additional ascorbate transporters in their cell membranes. These cells have a second defensive barrier against scurvy, since they can maintain high levels of ascorbate during times of shortage.

## Ascorbate transport

White blood cells transport ascorbate actively into their cell bodies. Ascorbate levels in these cells vary, covering a range from

25 to 80 times the levels in plasma. Neutrophils have an internal level of about 1.4 mM/L, other white cell types have higher levels (monocytes >3 mM/L, lymphocytes about 4 mM/L). Neutrophils therefore have the lowest vitamin C concentration of these cells.

White blood cells deplete, or lose their ascorbate, more slowly than other tissues, such as plasma and semen. Cells with slower depletion rates will retain ascorbate when other tissues are suffering from scurvy. The committee notes that repletion rates for white blood cells are faster than for other cells. This means that if there is a shortage of vitamin C, additional doses of ascorbate will top up the white blood cells preferentially, while other tissues are still deprived. This implies that the depletion-repletion studies of white blood cells do not model other tissues. The RDA committee ignored these important differences between white blood cells and other cells, thus their argument that neutrophils represent the whole body is flawed.

## Activated neutrophil transport

When an infection or invasion of microorganisms threatens the body, neutrophils become activated. In this activated state, they become phagocytic[W] and their ascorbate uptake mechanism differs from that in normal, non-phagocytic cells. Normally, neutrophils accumulate ascorbate directly.[72,73] However, when activated in inflammation or infection, neutrophils can increase their internal concentration of ascorbate by a factor of thirty,[74] which implies that neutrophil ascorbate absorption characteristics are specialised. The internal concentration of ascorbate, which is high even before activation, increases greatly when extra is needed. During activation, GLUT transporters pump the oxidised, dehydroascorbate (DHA) form of vitamin C into the cell, where it is reduced. In a healthy individual, the plasma concentration of dehydroascorbate should be low. However, neutrophils are unusual in that, when activated, they can oxidise ascorbate locally and transport the resulting DHA into the cell, before reducing it back to ascorbate.[75] The extent to which this indirect intake mechanism contributes to transport in un-activated neutrophils remains to be determined.

--------

[W] Phagocytic cells engulf bacteria and other foreign bodies.

Once again, there are problems with the NIH suggestions for saturation of neutrophils. The mechanisms used by neutrophils to absorb vitamin C are unusual. Despite this, the NIH would have us believe that neutrophils saturate in the same way as normal tissues. The glucose transporters (GLUT1 and GLUT3) in neutrophils have a similar affinity for glucose (Km ~ 1-5 mM) as they do for dehydroascorbate (Km ~ 1.1-1.7 mM). This means that the transporters pump glucose and dehydroascorbate at similar rates, when the concentrations are similar.[40,76] However, glucose is present in plasma at concentrations of 4-7 mM/L, which is up to 100 times higher than baseline ascorbate (~70 microM/L). In a healthy person, the ascorbate concentration is about 14-15 times that of dehydroascorbate.[48] This means the concentration of glucose is perhaps three orders of magnitude (or 1000 times) greater than that of dehydroascorbate, and could greatly inhibit the latter's uptake into typical cells.[40,61] Because of this, the contribution of these glucose transporters to vitamin C uptake by cells may be smaller than generally supposed.

## NIH white blood cell saturation

For some reason, the RDA committee used the NIH data on neutrophil white blood cells as their core data for the RDA. Dr Mark Levine from the NIH stated that he measured ascorbate levels in white blood cells for the sole reason that they were easy to sample.[77] On ethical grounds, he could not take biopsies of body tissues from healthy subjects. However, the researchers already had a supply of white blood cells, in the blood samples taken for the plasma measurements.

When we pointed out that white blood cells are highly specialised, especially for ascorbate absorption and biochemistry, Levine merely suggested that they might be a useful indicator for *some* other cells in the body. This is a reasonable and accurate statement. However, the extrapolation from the requirements of white blood cells to the whole body is unjustified. Red blood cells were also present in Levine's samples; these behave quite differently to white cells in their ascorbate absorption and internal concentration. However, the NIH experimenters did not investigate red blood cells.

## Why choose neutrophils?

The NIH did not consider the absorption characteristics of red blood cells, despite their ease of sampling. The properties of these cells are well described in the literature.[78,79,80,81,82,83] We are left to wonder whether the reason for this omission was simply because these cells do not saturate at a low dose but follow plasma levels.

Red blood cells could provide a more representative model than neutrophils for the wider system. Both red and white blood cells contain GLUT transporters that can absorb oxidised ascorbate. However, the concentration of ascorbate in red cells is much lower than that found in white blood cells. Red blood cells take in ascorbate slowly, by diffusion.[X] Despite the clear specialisation of red cells, their ascorbate uptake characteristics appear closer to the majority of body cells than do those of white cells.

Like typical body cells, red blood cells have a similar internal ascorbate concentration to the surrounding plasma. As the concentration in plasma increases, ascorbate diffuses into the red blood cells. However, at concentrations above the baseline, the rate of uptake by red cells is several times slower than the rate of excretion from plasma. A sustained increase in plasma concentration would be required to produce a consistent or maximal increase in red blood cell ascorbate concentration. Such a prolonged rise in plasma levels might greatly increase the internal concentration of these and other body cells. Red blood cell characteristics are clearly consistent with the dynamic flow model.

Despite the specialised and unrepresentative nature of white blood cells, the NIH measured levels of ascorbate in three white cell types: neutrophils, monocytes and lymphocytes. The RDA committee accept that ascorbate protects neutrophils and other white blood cells from oxidation damage during phagocytosis. From the cell types studied, the committee selected neutrophils. There was no explanation for this selection. We have noted that neutrophils had the lowest internal concentration,

---

[X] The intake rate has an inverse "half-life" of several hours.

which brought them closer to the much lower levels found in more typical tissues. This would minimise the discrepancy, but the concentration in neutrophils is still an order of magnitude too large.

## Oxidation

It is clear that the RDA committee are aware of the individual nature of the relationship between ascorbate and white blood cells, since they gave it a special section in their report.[7] They explained that the high content of vitamin C in white blood cells is especially important because these cells generate reactive oxygen species, such as superoxide and hydrogen peroxide. This synthesis of oxidants occurs when infection, inflammation and the presence of free radicals stimulate the activation of white blood cells. Typical body cells do not become activated or generate these high levels of oxidants.

Activated white blood cells, as the name suggests, have impressive biochemistry. When activated, isolated white blood cells increase ascorbate recycling by a factor of 30 compared to resting cells.[84] The ascorbate is recycled, oxidised to dehydroascorbate and re-reduced back to ascorbate, at a much higher rate. This process allows the white blood cells to neutralise the oxidants they form during phagocytosis. It is important to keep the white cell structures free from oxidation damage while the cell is destroying bacteria and other foreign bodies with oxidants.[66] The RDA committee accepts that ascorbate modulates the main physiological actions of activated white blood cells including phagocytosis, blastogenesis, antibody production and, possibly, chemotaxis and adhesiveness.[Y]

The committee suggests that a function of ascorbate is to neutralise the oxidant hypochlorous acid and to prevent protein damage at inflamed sites, such as arthritic joints. This effect occurs at levels normally found in plasma (22-85 microM/L), but higher levels could be more protective. They claim that the ratio of dehydroascorbate to ascorbate increases in inflamed sites, which is also a prediction of the dynamic flow model. The ratio of

---

[Y] Blastogenesis is when the cell multiplies by simple division, chemotaxis is movement of the cell towards a chemical stimulus.

oxidised to reduced ascorbate could be corrected by increasing the ascorbate concentration.[9] Along the same lines, the committee report increased oxidised ascorbate in the plasma of adult patients with respiratory distress syndrome, and in smokers. They also accept that the environmental pollutant ozone depletes ascorbate in the lung.

## Neutrophils need high plasma ascorbate levels

Even if neutrophils are used as a model for the body, the results indicate that high intakes are needed for optimal functioning. The RDA justification describes how superoxide production in neutrophils is inversely proportional to plasma ascorbate concentrations, within the range 22-85 microM/L. The RDA committee describes this range as normal. They claim that neutrophil superoxide production is lowered by 29%, 44%, 52% and 55% by extra-cellular concentrations of 28 microM/L, 57 microM/L, 114 microM/L and 284 microM/L respectively. This decrease in superoxide production had no reported effect on bactericidal killing. Thus, maximal plasma levels of ascorbate would reduce oxidative damage in these cells.

The committee go on to state:

"This indicates that antioxidant protection [for neutrophils] is increasingly provided as [plasma] ascorbate concentrations increase."

The committee therefore accepts that increasing the plasma ascorbate concentration provides increased protection against phagocyte-derived oxidant damage. This means that neutrophil function is dependent on high levels of ascorbate in plasma.

The increase in benefit continues up to 284 microM/L, which is above the steady state value of 220 microM/L, reached with an intake of 18 grams per day, in divided doses. The committee do not discuss the implication that optimal white blood cell functioning requires high steady state values for ascorbate in plasma. However, their own report suggests that optimal functioning of activated neutrophils requires high doses of ascorbate, in the dynamic flow range.

# Bias

The RDA committee's approach was biased and misleading; there is plenty of evidence to support this view in their publications. To begin with, let us examine some statements made by the committee:

> "...ascorbate at a physiologically relevant concentration of 50 microM/L (0.9mg/dl) was the most effective antioxidant for preventing LDL oxidation due to myeloperoxidase derived RNS."

The first problem with this statement is the term *physiologically relevant concentration*. 50 microM/L is a low blood level, and is below the baseline level of 70 microM/L. Although such low levels do occur physiologically, steady state levels with supplementation can be four to five times this concentration.

The second problem is that the committee do not specify which concentrations were compared to 50 microM/L, in deciding that it was the "most effective".[85] Since they did not state the range of concentrations studied, their statement is misleading. Also, the experiment was performed *in vitro* and extrapolation to the whole body is unjustified, without further evidence.

## Pre-selection of data

The RDA committee reveal their bias in the way they refer to experimental studies. For example, consider the following citation:

> "...in a recent review of epidemiological studies, Gey (1998) suggested that vitamin C concentrations as low as 50 microM/L (1.0mg/dl) provide the optimal benefits with regard to cardiovascular disease and cancer." [8,86]

Epidemiological studies involve populations that generally consume low levels of vitamin C. The committee suggests that a plasma level of 50 microM/L corresponds to an intake of 90mg per day. They add that Gey has suggested:

"...vitamin C concentrations as low as 50 microM/L provide the optimal benefits."

This is not true. The paper by Gey indicates that plasma levels *greater than or equal to 50 microM/L* are *desirable* for disease prevention. Gey does not use the term optimal, and the committee seem to have lost the greater than sign (>), which appears in Gey's paper.[z]

In addition to these factual inaccuracies, the use of epidemiological studies such as this can be criticised further. The dose range and plasma levels covered are restricted and do not include suitable numbers at the higher plasma levels. Such higher intakes are precisely those that are postulated to be most beneficial, for example, three grams or more in heart disease.[87,30,88,28,29] It is wrong to suggest that low intakes are optimal, as they have not been compared to the doses that are suggested to be protective. The committee does not have enough information to define an optimal dose, since there have not been enough studies of the effects of high doses.

Based on this evidence, the committee continues,

"...it may be difficult to do a large-scale trial that demonstrates a health benefit for vitamin C unless the subjects are pre-screened to have dietary intakes less than 90mg per day"

This loaded statement presents a shocking distortion of the facts. Gey's minimum level has now been represented as the maximum. Gey suggested a range of desirable plasma levels, with 50 microM/L as the lower limit. The committee members have taken Gey's minimum level and equated it to an intake of 90mg per day. They have then defined this minimum as "optimal". Since they have defined 90mg per day as the optimal intake, they apparently assume that studies above this level will not be beneficial. The minimum is now the maximum. *This is the exact opposite of the original findings.*

---

[z] They have assumed equality, ie =, rather than greater than or equals, ≥. Greater than or equals, ≥, becomes less than, <, in a classic case of doublethink.

Based on this faulty reasoning, the committee suggests pre-screening research subjects to have dietary intakes of less than 90mg per day, which would *prevent studies from finding the reported beneficial results of higher doses.* If scientists followed this guideline, there would be no studies on high dose vitamin C. This would prevent the very research that, according to the dynamic flow model and extensive clinical reports, would be most likely to show benefits.

Taken at face value, the RDA committee's pre-screening notion provides a justification for not supporting studies of higher doses in cardiovascular disease. In a wonderful example of circular logic, the committee uses studies that do not include high intakes to justify not studying high-dose supplements in the future. By misrepresenting the results, the committee excludes those doses that have been reported to show benefits. This would rule out clinical trials such as those based on the hypothesis that heart disease is a symptom of long-term ascorbate deficiency, which could be prevented or cured using high doses of vitamin C.

Until the theory that atherosclerosis is a kind of long-term scurvy has been refuted, the RDA is invalid. It remains possible that many people taking RDA level intakes will be catastrophically deficient in ascorbate. The responsibility for this deficiency rests with the RDA committee and their refusal to consider the full range of possible intakes. It is not sufficient to state that there is no compelling evidence for a theory, when the medical establishment has failed to carry out essential research.[9] Furthermore, it is unethical to ignore evidence for the role of higher doses when producing the RDA.

## Nutrition and pharmacology

The RDA committee accepts that supplementation with between 200mg and six grams of vitamin C per day has been shown to affect (in other words, improve) the functioning of the immune system. They equate these dose levels with pharmacology, rather than nutrition, stating that

> "...the results relate largely to the pharmacological range of vitamin C intakes rather than the nutritional range of intakes usually provided from food alone."

The purpose of the RDA committee is to determine the recommended nutritional doses and, in so doing, separate them from pharmacology. Their statement above pre-defines nutritional doses as those obtained from food alone. According to this, benefits from doses above those in the modern diet are pharmacological, by definition. So, supposing 500mg per day prevented heart disease, the result would have be deemed to have no importance to nutrition or to determination of the required intake, as the committee considers ascorbate at this dose to be a drug.

By indicating that a dose of 200mg is above the nutritional range, the RDA committee are pre-empting their conclusion. The quoted statement once again indicates that the committee had a pre-existing idea and range for nutritional doses; they have biased their recommendations according to their prejudice. We can also see the shadow of a further assumption: that the current modern diet, without supplementation, is adequate.

The idea that 200mg to six grams of vitamin C could not be obtained from the diet is incorrect. Linus Pauling estimated an intake of two and a half grams from raw fruit and vegetables; vegetarians might consume this amount from fresh organic produce.[10] Non-vegetarians could also obtain intakes above 200mg on a regular basis, depending on their diet.[AA]

The committee draw attention to variations in the results of studies of gram level supplementation, again indicating that improvements are not consistent. Some studies show benefits, some do not, although no studies demonstrate harm. The committee do not mention the timing of the doses, or the short half-life of the vitamin. They do not discuss the level of individual variation in response to supplementation. Furthermore, they fail to adequately describe the duration of the studies.

An optimal nutritional intake is the amount required each day for good health. Modern humans consume amounts that could be described as "nutritional" in the sense that they are taken, with other nutrients, in our normal food. However, independent

---

[AA] The oft-repeated recommendation that you should get all your vitamins from fruit and vegetables ignores the increasing loss of such nutrients in the breeding of plants for agriculture.

estimates of the optimal daily intake for vitamin C cover the range 200mg to 20 grams, depending on the individual.[9,38,10,48] To be clear, the minimum dose suggested by Linus Pauling and others, for prevention of heart disease, is three grams per day, in divided doses: Other scientists suggest higher doses, closer to bowel tolerance level, perhaps up to 20 grams per day. These high doses could be essential in people with a propensity for this disease.

The RDA committee has failed to explain how the low doses they propose could be optimal for cardiovascular health. Their report states that studies suggesting a protective effect against heart disease were insufficiently consistent or specific enough to indicate an RDA. This inconsistency is exactly what we would predict, if the doses under consideration were too low and too infrequent compared with those hypothesised to prevent heart disease.[9]

We should expect, however, that a committee with the responsibility for a decision affecting the health of millions would be sufficiently competent and open minded to evaluate all the available evidence. The reasons for the committee's apparent bias become clear when we consider the benefits of high doses.

# Benefits of high doses

For a cost-benefit analysis to be valid, both costs and benefits need to be addressed. In the case of the RDA, this requires an estimation of benefit across the range of doses. In this section, we demonstrate that the RDA committee have failed to take proper account of the benefits of higher doses.

The US committee claim the RDA is

"... the intake at which the risk of inadequacy is very small - only 0.02 to 0.03 (2% to 3%)." [8]

These values were derived using the "magical statistics" mentioned in the chapter on RDA Justification. The claimed risk of inadequacy is inaccurate and misleading, because the committee has ignored data on the benefits of higher doses. To quote the US RDA committee,

"The dietary allowances for vitamin C **must** be set, **somewhat arbitrarily**, between the amount necessary to prevent overt symptoms of scurvy (approximately 10mg/day in adults) and the amount beyond which the bulk of vitamin C is not retained in the body, but rather is excreted as such in the urine (approximately 200mg/day)." [7,BB]

This statement reveals the committee's prejudice, which has prevented it from carrying out an impartial evaluation of the data. The committee members assume that doses above 200mg are redundant, as they are not retained in the body. This is their justification for failing to consider the possibility of benefits arising from doses of more than 200mg/day. They ignore the benefits of intakes above 200mg, incorrectly assuming that such doses are purely pharmacological. The committee includes a few higher dose studies in its discussion, but does not consider these

---

[BB] Bold case added for emphasis.

studies pertinent to nutritional doses.[CC] Their statement admits setting the RDA "somewhat arbitrarily", thereby acknowledging that there is insufficient data upon which to base a recommendation. Many people might consider that to recommend a dietary intake for an entire population "somewhat arbitrarily" is unethical.

Here we list examples of positive effects the committee describes and then excludes as irrelevant to the RDA. We could fill several books with additional data, but refer the reader to existing sources.[9,38,48,10]

The UK expert committee are aware of the claimed benefits of higher doses; for example, they report that

> "There are many reports of vitamin C having beneficial effects in the healthy population at intakes and tissue levels considerably greater than those needed to prevent or treat scurvy." [2,5]

The US justification mentions several reports of benefits from high doses.[7] However, the listed positive reports represent only a small sample of the total available. Taken in isolation, the RDA documents give the misleading impression that few high dose studies indicate benefit. The absence of a comprehensive description of the claimed benefits of high doses weakens the RDA justification.

The RDA committee notes that vitamin C reduces oxidation in smokers. Oxidative stress increases with smoking and other activities that generate free radicals. The ratio of oxidised ascorbate (dehydroascorbate) to reduced ascorbate is increased in smokers, indicating oxidative stress.[89] Supplementation with two grams per day of ascorbate is claimed to decrease indicators of lipid peroxidation in smokers.[90] A dose of one gram per day lessens DNA damage in smokers by 20%.[91] The RDA committee agrees that supplementation with ascorbate at these gram level

---

[CC] This clear prejudice is a part of the establishment's nutritional paradigm and may explain how the NIH came to similar invalid conclusions in their pharmacokinetic studies.

doses "results in an antioxidant effect" that could be beneficial, especially in smokers.

The committee indicates that vitamin C decreases the oxidation of low density lipoprotein (LDL), also known as "bad" cholesterol, and that

"... the vitamin C supplements that resulted in positive effects ranged from 500mg to 2000mg per day."

LDL oxidation is a causative factor in atherosclerosis and heart disease. The RDA committee reports that LDL oxidation is inhibited by ascorbate concentrations above 40 microM/L. They describe 13 studies on biomarkers of LDL oxidation; seven of these used doses from 500mg to two grams, and showed positive results. The remaining studies used doses from 500mg to six grams, and showed no effect.

The committee provided evidence that ascorbate intake and plasma concentrations correlate with resistance to cardiovascular disease. The concentrations considered were in the range 11 microM/L (almost scurvy levels) to 153 microM/L (corresponding to gram level intake). Some studies did not show a benefit, so the committee described the results as inconsistent. It is important to add that the "negative" studies did not show harm. Given the short half-life of ascorbate, such mixed results are not surprising. Indeed, they are predicted by the dynamic flow model.[9] Despite the fact that the dosing regimes were far from optimal, more than half the studies reported showed that doses above 500mg were beneficial.

The committee describes these results as "inconclusive". This is an accurate statement, although the greater proportion of studies suggests a positive effect. A more balanced view might be that there is a reasonable indication that high doses of vitamin C inhibit LDL oxidation and reduce the possibility of atherosclerosis and its associated diseases, such as heart attack. In the absence of harmful effects, a cautious interpretation of these studies would be that the RDA should be at least 500mg per day.

The spacing of the supplementation in the reported experiments, whether given once or twice daily, is a likely explanation for the absence of positive effects in some of these

LDL oxidation studies. Because ascorbate has a short half-life, the blood level from a single dose above about 500mg does not differ from that of a single higher dose, in healthy people.[9] Within the half to six gram range studied, the plasma concentration would peak quickly and the levels would differ only briefly. After this time, the effects of the different doses would be the same. If the committee did not understand the implications of the short half-life of gram level doses, they could not be expected to appreciate that all the doses in these studies were equivalent, unless the dose was split into divided doses, given throughout the day. Divided doses produce a greater biological effect, as they raise the mean blood level more effectively.[9]

The committee reports that vitamin C supplementation (two grams per day) has an antioxidant effect in gastritis. In smokers, they report that the same dose increases plasma ascorbate levels and decreases the adhesion of monocyte white blood cells to endothelium. This adhesion process is involved in atherosclerosis and heart disease.

In the cancer biomarkers section of the RDA document, the committee considers a number of positive, higher-dose studies. Three studies out of five (doses 750mg – three grams) on patients with colorectal polyps were positive or showed no change, though the committee described the results as variable. Furthermore, supplementation with 1.5 grams ascorbate per day for one week reduced beta glucuronidase activity, a marker for cancer. For breast cancer, the reported studies (dose range 359-500mg) either gave positive results or showed no effect.

The committee report another high dose study, which found that doses of ascorbate of 490mg per day have a protective effect against cataracts. Lower doses of ascorbate, less than 260mg per day, were not effective.

In discussing the common cold, the committee acknowledge the existence of Linus Pauling and the hypothesis that megadoses of ascorbate may be preventative. Although well known, this is perhaps the least important of Pauling's claims for vitamin C. The results for the common cold were confusing but are also consistent with a large protective and treatment effect. Once again, the dynamic flow model explains this variation in results as a consequence of the short half-life of higher doses. The variability in the results of these methodologically flawed studies is consistent with the suggestion that high doses of ascorbate given as frequent, split doses are likely to be more effective than single daily doses.[9]

The RDA committee's recommendations are one-sided: they do not consider the risks to the population of losing the benefits that might be gained from higher, properly spaced, doses of vitamin C.

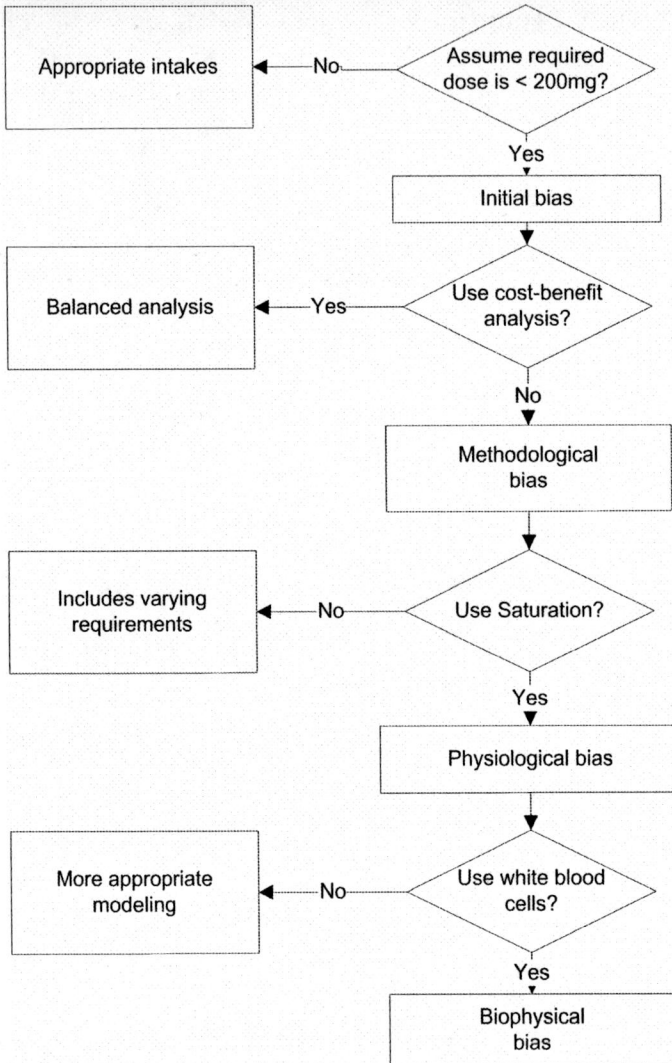

RDA
Introduction of bias

Appropriate intakes ◄—No— Assume required dose is < 200mg?

Yes
Initial bias

Balanced analysis ◄—Yes— Use cost-benefit analysis?

No
Methodological bias

Includes varying requirements ◄—No— Use Saturation?

Yes
Physiological bias

More appropriate modeling ◄—No— Use white blood cells?

Yes
Biophysical bias

# Costs and benefits

Neither the US nor the UK committees applied any form of optimisation technique in developing their recommendations. Such an approach would have minimised bias in their recommendations. In many scientific disciplines, it would be considered reckless to attempt to define an optimised value, such as the RDA, without use of a formal strategy.

As it stands, the RDA is based on risk assessment, with little regard for potential benefits. Imagine such a risk analysis performed on air travel, without consideration of the benefits. Since aeroplanes occasionally crash, the risk of death would ground all air transport. People are willing to accept the small risks associated with air travel because of the benefits of speed and cost, compared with other forms of travel. The actual risk is low and people might be at greater peril using alternative methods of transport.

The optimal intake of ascorbate depends on a small number of factors. On the cost side, these include the probability of side effects and the financial costs of the vitamin. The health costs of too high or too low a recommended dose are also relevant. On the benefits side, we need to consider the reduction in disease offered by different doses, together with the possible health care cost savings.

**Value of dose = Estimated benefit - Estimated harm**

In the case of vitamin C, the estimated harm is negligible. For this reason, the optimal intake approximates to the highest intake that can be shown to provide additional benefit.

Below, we summarise the data relating to the costs and benefits of vitamin C supplementation.

## Costs

### Toxicity

The potential for harmful effects from ascorbate is low for the whole range of doses, up to the bowel tolerance level. Indeed, there is insufficient data to suggest that a dose of, say, 10 grams is more toxic than a dose of 500mg. In the words of the UK expert committee,[3]

> "The available data suggest that vitamin C is not associated with significant adverse effects and there are no obvious specific key toxic endpoints for vitamin C dose given orally to healthy subjects."

In pharmacology, there is a general heuristic that side effects are proportional to the dose. We can assume that higher intakes are more likely to reveal side effects than lower intakes. However, for a healthy adult with an ascorbate intake below the bowel tolerance level, there are only unsubstantiated, theoretical suggestions of toxicity.

### Financial costs

The cost of supplementing with a few grams of ascorbate per day is low. The cost difference between a 100mg and a 1000mg supplement may be negligible.

On the other hand, the financial cost of a degenerative disease or heart attack caused by insufficient intake may be catastrophic for the individual, substantial for the health services and profitable for doctors and drug companies.

## Benefits

The UK expert committee accepts that studies have reported beneficial effects on conditions such as cancer, vascular disease, cataracts, diabetes, asthma, arthritis, Parkinson's disease, autism and depression. However, they claim that these effects are not nutritional.[3] Unfortunately, the medical establishment has avoided research in this area to a degree that could be interpreted as deliberate suppression.[9] Despite this, substantial evidence from clinical trials, *in vitro* and *in vivo* experimental studies, physiological and biochemical research indicates benefits from high doses. With ultra high doses, there are few, if any, refutations and decades of clinical reports.[9,11]

The US RDA committee has tried to dismiss studies of high dose ascorbate by asserting that the dose is pharmacological; this claim needs to be demonstrated, however. Ascorbate kills cancer cells and leaves normal cells unharmed. Some scientists believe that atherosclerosis, heart disease and stroke are a result of chronically inadequate ascorbate intake, which needs to be at gram levels in susceptible individuals. There have been multiple observations of benefit in shock, infection, arthritis and other degenerative diseases. In the face of this evidence and the absence of demonstrable toxicity, the committee is taking a great risk by limiting daily intake to levels that prevent acute scurvy. While the RDA committees may believe their recommendations to be conservative, the cost-benefit analysis reveals them as foolhardy to the point of recklessness.

## The US RDA

The following table shows the dose and benefits from studies in the US RDA justification document:

| Intake (mg) | Benefit | Quality[DD] |
|:-----------:|:--------|:-----------:|
| 490 | Protective against cataracts | + |
| 1000 | Reduced DNA damage (smokers) | + |
| 2000 | Antioxidant effect in gastritis | + |
| 2000 | Reduced lipid peroxidation (smokers) | + |
| 500-2000 | Biomarkers of LDL oxidation | ++ (7/13) |
| 750-3000 | Colorectal polyps | + |

---

[DD] The subjective quality of the data is indicated reasonable + or good ++.

From this data, the minimum daily intake that provides nutritional benefit is about 500mg per day.[EE] There is no evidence of toxicity at this dose.

We remind the reader of three core questions:

- What benefits do the data suggest?

- What dose was used to achieve this benefit?

- How important is the benefit, relative to the known toxicity at this dose?

### Suggested benefits

The benefits listed by the committee are a tiny subset of those available. While we could list hundreds of studies, covering a range of diseases, we will just consider some additional factors for heart disease and mortality. These extend the results for lipid/LDL oxidation in the above table.

In a brief review for the Life Extension Foundation, Dr Paul Wand found 30 studies showing benefit (with four showing no benefit) in atherosclerosis, with intakes above 500mg. Intakes below 500mg were not effective, as predicted by the dynamic flow model.[9] In a study of 85,118 women, vitamin C supplementation reduced the risk of heart disease by 28%.[92] There are thousands of deaths each year from heart disease and cancer. Older people in the UK with low levels of vitamin C (<17 microM/L) have double the death rate of those with levels at plasma baseline or above (>67 microM/L).[93] It is claimed that in the US, men with the lowest blood levels (<28 microM/L) had a 57% higher risk of dying from any cause and a 62% higher risk of dying from cancer compared to men with the highest levels (>73 microM/L), though there was no increase in heart disease mortality.[94] In 6,624 US adults, lower vitamin C in plasma was associated with increased heart disease and stroke.[95]

In 2001, 19,496 people aged 45-79 years were studied for four years, to determine the effect of ascorbate on mortality.[96] In

---

the people taking most ascorbate, the risk of dying was only half that of those with the lowest intakes. The relationship between ascorbate and mortality was continuous through the whole range of intakes. A 20 microM/L rise in plasma ascorbate was associated with a 20% reduction in mortality from all causes. Over a period of more than half a century, several researchers have suggested that shortage of ascorbate in the diet is the *primary* cause of heart disease.[97,98,99,100,28,29] During the editing of this book, a pooled analysis of nine prospective studies was published. The analysis indicated that a dose of 700mg per day of ascorbate would reduce the risk of major coronary heart disease events by 25%. This figure is from a ten-year follow-up of 4,647 major coronary events in 293,172 subjects who had apparently healthy hearts at the start of the study.[101] However, data from clinical trials of vitamin C as a treatment for heart disease is limited,[102] as such research has been denigrated for over half a century.

### Dose used to achieve this benefit

In these cardiovascular studies, doses above 500mg per day were beneficial. Above this intake, single doses give similar blood profiles. The 500mg dose in these experiments represents a single daily dose, although multiple daily doses may provide additional benefit. If independent doses 24 hours apart provide benefit, then shortening the dose interval is likely to provide more benefit than giving a larger, single dose.[9] Some individuals, including the stressed or sick, may require much greater doses.

### Importance of benefit, relative to known toxicity

There is reasonable evidence of benefit with little, if any, identifiable health cost. The plasma response for 500mg is comparable to that for higher intakes, assuming the person is healthy, so a 500mg dose will provide similar benefits while minimising any possible risk. Based on the suggested benefits, we conclude that the minimum possible value for the RDA is 500mg, with the caveat that frequent, repeated doses of this size are more likely to be beneficial.

## RDA conclusions

Even the US recommendation of 90mg per day is likely to leave people chronically deficient. However, the UK RDA is lower than the US value. We note that intakes of 30-60mg are considered marginal by some authors.[103] People consuming the current UK recommendation of 40mg per day may be putting themselves at risk of severe disease in the longer term. This intake will prevent acute scurvy, but may leave people susceptible to chronic illnesses.

## Dynamic flow

The questions of benefits and toxicity are the same for dynamic flow as with the US RDA value, and are not repeated here. This section considers specific aspects of the dynamic flow dosing regime.

The RDA is generally expressed as a daily intake, without regard to the dosing regimen. This simplistic approach is inappropriate, because of the way the body uses vitamin C. Any estimate of requirements should take into account the two-phase plasma pharmacokinetics of ascorbate. Below the plasma baseline, pumps in the kidneys retain ascorbate to protect the body pool. Above the baseline, the short half-life of ascorbate (0.5 hours) means that *no estimate of requirements should ignore the number and timing of intakes*. The RDA committee have ignored the possibility of benefits from doses leading to levels above the plasma baseline.

The dynamic flow model predicts that single daily dose studies will grossly underestimate any observed benefits.[9] To be clear, let us consider a dose of three grams per day. The model implies that six half-gram doses taken at four hourly intervals will be therapeutically more effective than a daily dose of three grams taken at one time. Dividing the dose in this way would not increase the known toxicity, rather the reverse, because the smaller individual doses are likely to fall below bowel tolerance levels.

The three core questions above lead directly to dynamic flow, as the preferred method and level of intake. In healthy, young adults, according to the dynamic flow model, amounts of 500mg or more, taken several times a day, can allow a steady state, close to "saturation", with some unabsorbed reserve. This means that a daily intake of 2-3 grams, in divided doses, can provide many of the benefits of plasma saturation, for a minimal dose.

# Quantifiable biomarkers for scurvy

The optimal nutritional intake is the amount required each day for good health. As we have seen, independent estimates of the optimal intake for ascorbate vary from 200mg to 20 grams each day.[9,38,10,11,48] The minimum dose suggested by Linus Pauling and others, for prevention of heart disease, is three grams per day, in divided doses. Several other scientists suggest much higher doses, closer to bowel tolerance level. These high doses may be essential in susceptible individuals, to prevent disease.

One of the main difficulties for the RDA committees seems to be finding an adequate measure of ascorbate requirements. We therefore suggest some alternative possibilities. [FF]

The first method we suggest is physiological: the use of bowel tolerance in the individual. Bowel tolerance may be used as a measure of individual need, as suggested by Dr Robert Cathcart. This suggestion is entirely consistent with the committee's use of bowel tolerance as an indicator of the tolerable upper limit. Application of the upper limit approach to individuals, rather than the whole population, allows for biological variation. This is consistent with the modern medical model.

Secondly, we suggest that red blood cells, as opposed to white blood cells as used for current RDAs, may provide a more appropriate model for typical body tissues. These red cells are easy to sample and are more representative of the wider body tissues.

The third technique is new, and depends on the action of ascorbate on blood vessels. The effect of vitamin C on damaged blood vessels on the retina can be measured. Images of the retina and its blood vessels are taken routinely at optometry clinics. Optometrist Dr Sydney Bush has proposed a new technique,

---

[FF] We are not proposing a new RDA but suggesting that intake can be ultimately derived using rigorous methods.

which he calls CardioRetinometry, for estimation of vitamin C requirements.

The reported action of ascorbate on the pericorneal blood vessels is both striking and quantifiable. It is similar to the action of epinephrine, and suggests an important effect of high dose ascorbate on the cardiovascular system.

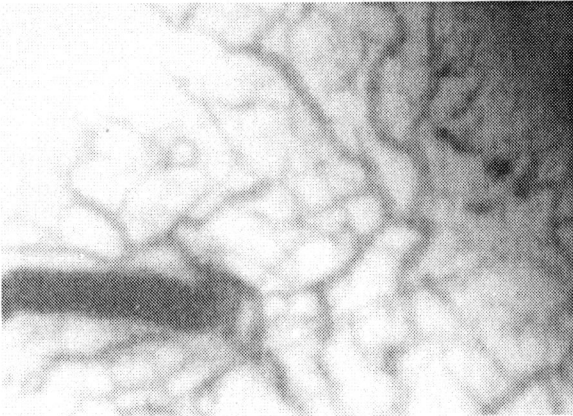

Initial pericorneal image from subject showing indications of mild inflammation note the small aneurisms in the centre right of the image.

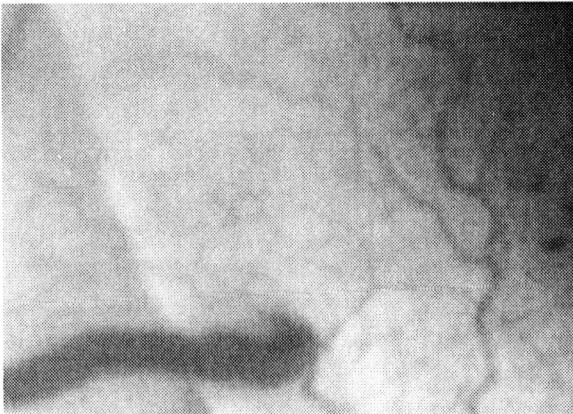

Pericornea following oral megadose ascorbate for one week, showing improvement to the microvasculature.

The action of oral vitamin C on the microvasculature may be quantifiable. This effect may provide a measure for a more rigorous derivation of intake requirements.

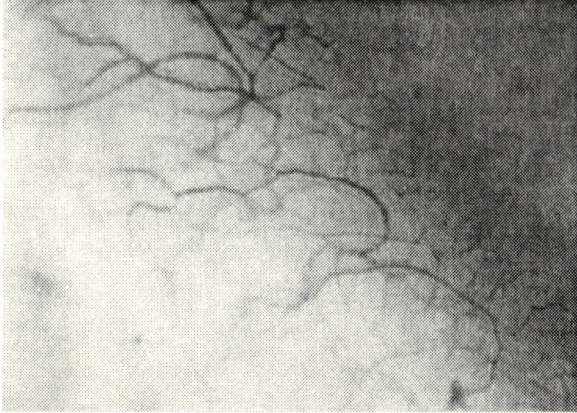

This first image of the pericornea shows retinal blood vessels before administration of ascorbate. Note the degree of blood vessel swelling.

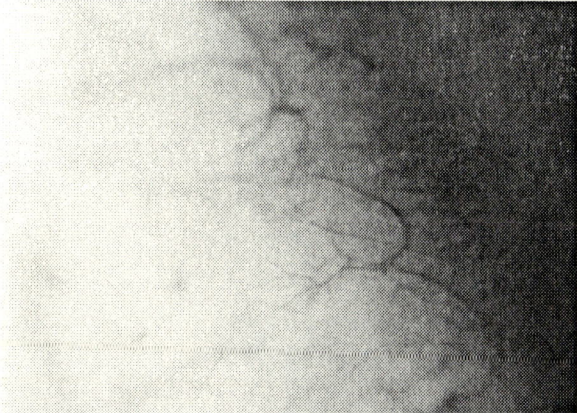

After only one week of megadose vitamin C, the previously enlarged blood vessels have constricted, producing an improved appearance to the pericornea. Compare the aneurisms, or small swellings in the blood vessels, with those in the original image.

Over a number of years, Dr Bush made observations on about 1000 patients attending his eye clinic. In retinal examination, he successfully imaged the small blood vessels, which provide a window on the state of the vasculature within the body. Changes and micro-aneurisms in blood vessels are suggestive of hypertension, stroke and cardiovascular disease.[104,105,106,107,108,109,110,111,112] In particular, the ratio of arteriolar to venular diameter may be used as an indicator of pathological processes. Narrowed retinal arterioles are associated with a long-term risk of hypertension, suggesting that structural alterations of the microvasculature may be linked to the development of hypertension.[112] Bush found reductions of blood vessel lumen, congestion and increased blood in the tissue, called hyperaemia, in almost every apparently normal adult subject he examined. He generated the theory that scurvy was leading to blood vessel damage. He made a preliminary redefinition of scurvy as:

"any state in which supplemental vitamin C improves the pericorneal vasculature"[113]

According to Bush, sub-clinical scurvy is any intake below the minimum necessary to produce healthy blood vessels in the eye. This potentially provides a qualitative and quantitative method, based on elementary image analysis,[114,115,116,117] for the determination of vitamin C requirements. While it applies only to microvascular health, this approach is potentially a practical, low cost measure of ascorbate requirements.

The method requires validation and clinical trials, but may lead the way to a quantitative method of assessing scurvy in humans. Bush has been using a semi-quantitative observational grading technique to evaluate the images.

Bush claims to have treated patients with ascorbate over several years. He found that micro-aneurysms, or bulging of small arteries caused by weakening of the artery wall, were gradually eliminated as ascorbate intake increased. He estimated that retinal blood vessels improved in over 90% of patients taking high dose ascorbate. Measurement of such blood vessels seems to be reliable but the response of an individual will vary with time.[118] Bush also claims that cholesterol deposits in the retina become smaller and are reversed, in the longer term. This observation is consistent with the claims of Pauling and others for heart disease as scurvy. Bush's results require independent confirmation. Notably, however, some subjects needed over 10 grams per day, together with vitamin E, for the full effect. This intake is more than 100 times the RDA.

We must consider the limitations of these current results. The objections to Bush's work include lack of randomised, double-blind controls, and potential observer bias. However, the change in the retinal blood vessels observed by Bush is described as much larger than normal variation and equivalent to the action of epinephrine. We consider that image selection appears to be a more productive objection than the placebo effect. However, Bush reports a consistent and large effect, which is easily replicable in a short period by an independent experimenter at low cost. Objections to this work carry little weight, as such replication could produce a definitive refutation.

# RDA
## Reducing bias

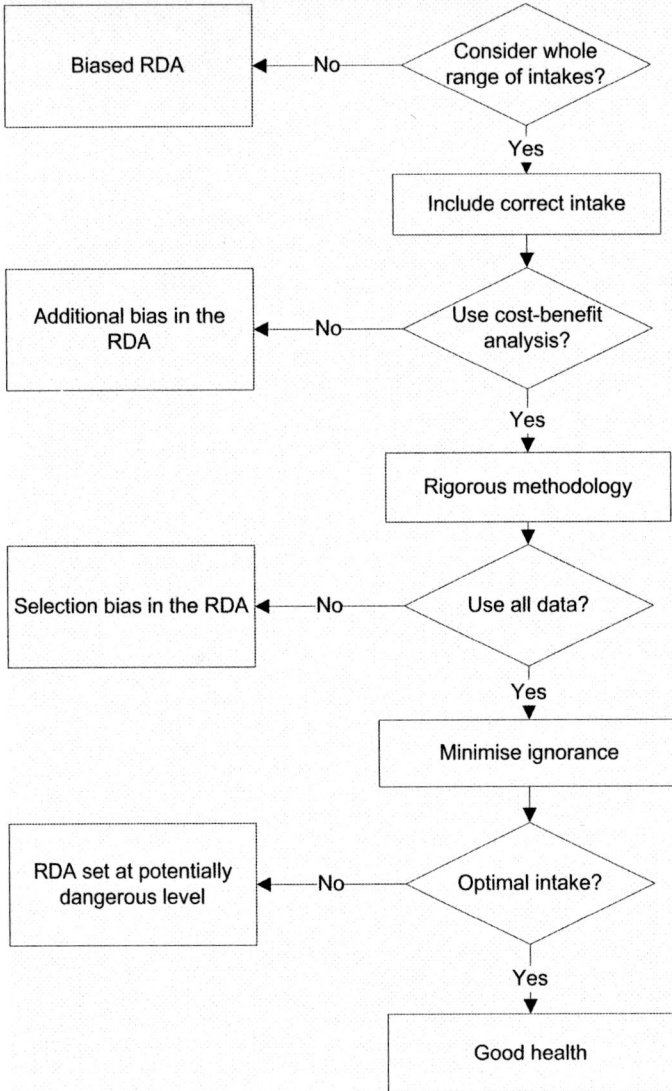

| | | |
|---|---|---|
| **Biased RDA** | ◀— No — | Consider whole range of intakes? |

Yes ▼

Include correct intake

▼

| | | |
|---|---|---|
| **Additional bias in the RDA** | ◀— No — | Use cost-benefit analysis? |

Yes ▼

Rigorous methodology

▼

| | | |
|---|---|---|
| **Selection bias in the RDA** | ◀— No — | Use all data? |

Yes ▼

Minimise ignorance

▼

| | | |
|---|---|---|
| **RDA set at potentially dangerous level** | ◀— No — | Optimal intake? |

Yes ▼

Good health

# Refutation

We hope you have enjoyed this refutation of the Ridiculous Dietary Allowance. It should be clear why the name was changed from Recommended Dietary Allowance to something more appropriate. In the *Ascorbate* book,[9] we invited readers to review the supporting evidence for the RDA critically, as it could hardly be described as scientific. Here, we have gone a little further and openly challenge this RDA nonsense.

We know many educated people who assume that nutrients at RDA levels are scientifically optimal. We have often been told that higher doses can be dangerous. Governments urge us to believe that we can get all the vitamins needed from five helpings of fruit and vegetables. Based on the evidence, we believe the public has been actively misled. Despite this, the sales of vitamin C supplements continue and many people regard Linus Pauling's recommendations more highly than they do government publications.

In the UK, the committee accept that the optimal intake of ascorbate is unknown.[2] Since this lack of knowledge is accepted, we cannot but wonder how the government can recommend a low value of 40mg,[5] when a suboptimal amount could result in ill health and premature death. They do not discuss the risks involved in underestimating the dose. At a daily intake of 83.4 mg, almost twice the recommended intake, the expert committee estimate that half the population will have plasma concentrations of 50 microM/L, which is below baseline levels. The elderly and smokers need higher intakes (150.2mg and 206.6mg, respectively) to achieve even this deficient state.[2]

The Linus Pauling Institute (LPI) has based its recommendation on the flawed NIH data. This recommendation differs greatly from that of Pauling himself. Presumably, when the NIH published their erroneous research, they provided an opportunity for the LPI to become more acceptable to the establishment. There is a practical side to this, as unless the Institute is valued by establishment scientists, government research funding might not be forthcoming. Unlike the NIH scientists, Dr Balz Frei, Director of the LPI, was willing to engage in discussion of the supporting evidence for the low-dose hypothesis. I think it is fair to say that we were able to counter his arguments and data. Despite this, the LPI will be retaining their "middle ground" recommendation of 400mg per day, until the establishment have acknowledged that a revision of the RDA is required. Readers may think Pauling would be disappointed with this timid approach by the institute that bears his name. However, at least the institute's director has been willing to go over the evidence in a scientific manner.

The Institute of Medicine claim they based their 90mg per day RDA on scientific principles. However, they apparently have no mechanism to deal with new scientific findings and seem to believe it is not necessary to defend their recommendations. We find their published justification, and that of their UK expert committee counterparts, to be based on prejudice, bias and conjecture.

## Scientific suppression

One of the conclusions of the RDA committee is that studies at or above the point where the body tissues are "saturated" may obscure the possible relationships between vitamin C intake and disease risk. This argument could be considered a way of preventing or suppressing research into high doses. If the body were genuinely saturated, there would be no point in studying higher dose supplements.

The RDA committee's conclusions include the idea that research should be conducted into finding possible adverse effects of high doses. This seems reasonable, but ignores the evidence for the benefits of high doses. They propose a guide to future research that avoids searching for benefits for high doses (above 90mg per day), but actively searches for side effects. This bias reveals muddled thinking. In their view, the body is saturated at 200mg, so there should be no point looking for benefits at higher doses. They do not appear to realise that if the body were really saturated at this low dose, higher doses would not produce side effects, for the same reason they would not provide benefits: the dose would not be absorbed.[GG] It is irrational to propose that an unabsorbed dose can cause kidney stones.

Their argument is not an unbiased cost-benefit analysis, but a suggestion to promote further selective research, with potentially dangerous consequences for the health of the population.

The medical establishment was arrogant enough to ignore and belittle Pauling's suggestions for higher doses. A small cabal of scientists, centred on the NIH and Institute of Medicine in the United States together with the Scientific Advisory Committee on Nutrition and the EVM committee in the UK, are responsible for promoting medicine's infatuation with low doses. The total number of scientists involved is small, but the influence they command is substantial.

## Requirement to explain

We were driven to write this book because the NIH and US RDA committee were unwilling to defend their conclusions. We do not understand this attitude. Scientists have a duty to explain and defend their ideas. This is not an academic exercise, as the health of millions depends on their ideas and recommendations.

One of our reviewers suggested that we tone down the comments in this book to something more acceptable to the government scientists involved. It is possible that by making the arguments more palatable to the authorities, we might stand a better chance of converting them to a more scientific approach. However, people have been trying to persuade the establishment to carry out a proper evaluation of ascorbate and other nutrients for many decades. Providing evidence for the benefits of high doses would not work, as such doses would be dismissed as "pharmacological". The flaws in the science needed to be made apparent. We felt obliged to point out the gross limitations in the current establishment science, which purports to support the RDA.

---

[GG] There would, however, be the possibility of gut-related side effects because of the higher local concentration with the increased dose.

We have described the failure of this establishment science in direct terms. The establishment claim to know the amount required for people each day, based on scientific evidence. This has continued for many years, ignoring the direct challenge of eminent scientists such as Linus Pauling. Many people believe that recommending low intakes of vitamin C places the health of the population at risk and could result in many premature deaths. This book was necessary. The errors, omissions and bias in the RDA and tolerable upper limits need to be made clear.

We are not proposing an intake level for ascorbate; there is insufficient data on which to base such a recommendation. However, it seems clear that doses of ascorbate should be spread throughout the day, because of the short half-life. The minimum dose to approach the maximum steady-state plasma value and allow dynamic flow would be three grams per day, taken in divided doses of 500mg. This estimate can be derived quantitatively from plasma values. It is explicitly not realistic for the whole population, as people are likely to vary in their requirements: sick people require much more.

The people claiming to have established the required intake are reluctant to defend their recommendations. Presumably, they think the population should take their advice automatically. It does not matter that they cannot provide a consistent justification, or that there is no mechanism to change the advice quickly, if new results show it to be wrong. They do not seem to realise that millions of people will die if they underestimate the intake. For them, evidence is selective and can be ignored. The RDA is not science, it is politics.

## Open challenge

We can find no scientific or even rational reasons for the current RDA values. The published justifications show clear and unambiguous bias. This bias could arise from peer pressure, ignorance, or corruption. We prefer the explanation that the people setting the RDA are honest and competent professionals, who were acting on a misleading and incorrect interpretation of the available data. If we are correct about the origin of the bias, we should expect them to be willing to review their current proposals. If the RDA recommendations are genuine, they should be defended in open scientific debate. As far as we can see, the reluctance to engage in open discussion with independent nutritional scientists suggests that the RDA is not scientifically viable.

The low intake RDA values require an explanation. If the RDA values have any scientific standing, it is as hypotheses. These hypotheses must be stated simply and clearly, and the critical supporting evidence should be indicated. The primary reason for the recommended intake should be easy to describe in a paragraph or two, citing the research papers that indicate that this dose is optimal.

We suggest this paragraph begins:

"The reason for recommending that an intake of X mg per day is optimal is..."

Supporting references should provide evidence that is specific, consistent and compelling, just as the RDA committee required of the high dose research. Unless such a statement is forthcoming, we assert that the current low dose RDA model for ascorbate should be abandoned.

A similar statement is required for the tolerable upper limit. Likewise, each nutrient for which governments or the Codex proposes an RDA or upper limit requires a simple statement of scientific justification that is independently validated.

We challenge the RDA committees and the Codex experts to provide such statements, for independent verification.

# Appendix A

## A PLEA FOR SCIENTIFIC RE-EVALUATION OF THE RECOMMENDED DIETARY ALLOWANCE FOR VITAMIN C

The following letter was organised by Bill Sardi:
August 23, 2004

Linda D. Meyers, PhD
Director, Food & Nutrition Board
Institute of Medicine
500 Fifth Street NW
Washington, DC 20001
Tel: 202.334.3153 Fax: 202.334.1412
Email: lmeyers@nas.edu

Catherine Woteki, PhD
Chair, Food & Nutrtion Board
Dean and Director, Department of Food Science and Human Nutrition
Iowa State Univ., College of Agriculture
138 Curtiss Hall
Ames, Iowa 50011
Phone: 515 294-2518
Fax: 515 294-6800
Email agdean@iastate.edu

Paul M. Coates, PhD
Director
Office of Dietary Supplements
National Institutes of Health
Suite 3B01, MSC 7517
6100 Executive Boulevard
Bethesda, Maryland 20892-7517
Fax: 301 480-1845
Email: ds@nih.gov

Senator Thomas Harkin
Attention to: Peter Reinecke,
Chief of staff
731 Hart Senate Office Building
Washington, DC 20510
Phone: (202) 224-3254
Fax: (202) 224-9369
tom_harkin@harkin.senate.gov

# PLEA CONCERNING ORAL VITAMIN C/RDA FOR VITAMIN C

As health professionals who have been involved in vitamin C research, it has recently come to our attention that higher blood plasma concentrations of vitamin C can be achieved through oral intake than previously thought possible. This scientific revelation has ramifications upon the current Recommended Dietary Allowance for vitamin C and personal health regimens for consumers. It is apparent the current published advice, that the blood plasma concentration for vitamin C is saturated at 200 milligrams oral consumption, must be revised. Furthermore, it is apparent the RDA for vitamin C needs immediate re-evaluation. We urge the scientific community and other responsible health authorities to take timely action to correct misinformation concerning oral dosing of vitamin C and to join an effort to re-evaluate the RDA for vitamin C.

Signed:

Steve Hickey Ph.D., Metropolitan University of Manchester, England. Co-author, Ascorbate, The Science of Vitamin C.

Hilary Roberts, Ph.D., graduate University of Manchester, England.

Professor Ian Brighthope, Managing Director, Nutrition Care Pharmaceuticals Pty Ltd, 25 - 27 Keysborough Avenue, Keysborough Victoria 3173 Australia.

Robert F. Cathcart III, M.D., practicing physician, advocate of high-dose vitamin C therapy; 127 Second Street, Suite 4, Los Altos, California 94022.

Abram Hoffer, M.D., PhD., F.R.C.P. ; Editor-in-chief of the Journal of Orthomolecular Medicine; Suite 3 - 2727 Quadra St ; Victoria, British Columbia V8T 4E5 Canada.

Patrick Holford, London, founder of the Institute for Optimum Nutrition (ION) and the Brain Bio Centre; author of The Optimum Nutrition Bible.

Dr Archie Kalokerinos, M.D., Graduate Sydney University. He is a Life Fellow of the Royal Society for Health, a Fellow of the International Academy of Preventive Medicine, Fellow of the Australasian College of Biomedical Scientists, and a Member of the New York Academy of Sciences. He has authored Vitamin C: Nature's Miraculous Healing Missile (1993). Currently he is semi-retired, living in Tamworth, New

South Wales. Address: 20 Kennedy Close, Cooranbong, Australia, NSW 2265.

Thomas Edward Levy, M.D., J.D., Tulane University School of Medicine, 1972-76-M.D.; Fellowship in Cardiology, 1979-81, Tulane University Affiliated Hospitals; author, "Vitamin C, Infectious Diseases, and Toxins".

Dr. Richard A. Passwater, Ph.D., antioxidant researcher, author "Supernutrition," Berlin, Maryland.

Hugh D. Riordan, M.D., President - The Center for the Improvement of Human Functioning Int'l, Inc., Director - Bio-Communications Research Institute, 3100 North Hillside Avenue, Wichita, KS 67219 U.S.A.

Andrew W. Saul, PhD, Contributing Editor, Journal of Orthomolecular Medicine, Number 8 Van Buren Street, Holley, New York 14470 USA.

Knowledge of Health, Inc.
457 West Allen Avenue #117 San Dimas, Ca. 91773 USA

# Appendix B

Members of the UK expert committee on the safety of vitamins and minerals (EVM), from the UK Government's Food Standards Agency website. Responsible for recommending the tolerable upper limit in the UK.

Chairman
**Professor M J S Langman** BSc, MD, FRCP, University of Birmingham, Birmingham
Members
**Professor P Aggett** OBE, MB, ChB, FRCP, MSC, DCH University of Central Lancashire, Preston
**Professor D S Davies** BSc, PhD, CChem, FRSC, FRCP, FRC Path. Imperial College School of Medicine, London
**Professor A A Jackson** BA, MBBCHIR, MD, FRCP University of Southampton, Southampton
**Professor B J Kirby** OBE, MB, ChB, FRCP, FRCPEd University of Exeter, Exeter
**Professor A E McLean** BM, BCh, PhD, FRCPath University College, London
**Professor A G Renwick** OBE, BSc, PhD, DSc University of Southampton, Southampton
**Dr L Rushton** BA, MSc, PhD, CStat MRC Institute for Environment and Health, Leicester
**Ms B Saunders** OBE, BA Independent Consumer Consultant, St Albans, Herts
**Ms C E Shaw** BSc, SRD The Royal Marsden NHS Trust, London
**Dr A J Thomas** PhD, FRCP, MB, ChB Plymouth Hospitals NHS Trust and Peninsula Medical School Universities of Exeter and Plymouth
**Dr A F Williams** BSc, MB, BS, D.Phil, FRCP, FRCPCH St Georges Hospital Medical School, London

## Declaration of Interests

The pharmaceutical and medical industries might expect to gain financially if the Tolerable Upper Limit for vitamin C and other nutrients is set at a suboptimal level. By definition, a suboptimal intake for the population will result in a reduction in health, the possibility of increased illness and increased drug sales. A commercial interest in a drug company is a conflict of interest. Such an interest might prohibit membership of the EVM committee to prevent possible bias. However, in the UK committee such commercial interests are extensive. The reader is invited to decide for themselves if they think these financial interests are desirable.

| Member | Personal Interests | | Other Interests | |
|---|---|---|---|---|
| | Company | Nature | Company | Nature |
| Michael Langman | None | | Merck Sharp & Dohne Boots Pharmaceuticals Astra Zeneca | All these refer to research support and collaborations |
| Peter Aggett | Nestlé Unilever Borax | Lecture Fees Lecture Fees Lecture Fees | DSM-GB Meat and Livestock Commission Abbot Roche Numicon | All these refer to support for departmental research or consultancy |
| Donald Davies | ICI Plc Astrazeneca PLC SKB Servier Lab ML Laboratories | Shareholding Shareholding Consultancy Consultancy Executive Director | Astrazeneca Bayer Plc Bristol Myers Squibb Curis (USA) Glaxo Wellcome Lilly Research Merck Sharp & Dohme ML Laboratories Orion-Farmos Pfizer Rhone-Poulenc Rorer Roche Sanofi Winthrop Schwarz Pharma Servier Smithkline Beecham Solvay | All of these interests relate to either commissioned research, meeting support or advisory work |
| Alan Jackson | None | | Vitaflo Hoffman la Roche Unilever Nutricia Research Foundation | Research support Research support Research support Research Support |
| Brian Kirby | None | | None | |

| André McLean | Smith & Nephew Ltd | Consultancy | | |
| | 3M Pharmaceuticals | Consultancy | | |
| | Glaxo Wellcome | Shareholding | | |
| | Brittania Pharmaceuticals | Commissioned work | | |
| | Charterhouse Clincal Research Ltd | Commissioned work | | |
| | Galen Pharmaceuticals Ltd | Commissioned work | | |
| | Esteve Pharmaceticals, Spain | Commissioned work | | |
| | Omrix Pharmaceuticals | Commissioned work | | |
| | Ajinomoto Pharmaceuticals | Commissioned work | | |
| Andrew Renwick | International Sweeteners Association | Consultant | Hoffman-La Roche | Research support |
| | Neste | Fee for writing an Expert Opinion | SmithKline Beecham | Research support |
| | | | Pfizer | Research support |
| | | | Flavour and Extract Manufacturers Association (FEMA) | Research support |
| | | | American Chemistry Council | Research support |
| | | | | Research support |
| Lesley Rushton | None | | None | |
| Barbara Saunders | None | | None | |
| Clare Shaw | Novartis Consumer Health | Fee for writing/editing publication | None | |
| Anita Thomas | None | | None | |
| Anthony Williams | None | | None | |

125

# Appendix C

US Food and Nutrition Board Members from the Institute of Medicine's website are listed here. These are the experts directly responsible for justifying the US RDA.

**Catherine E. Woteki, Ph.D., R.D.** *(chair),* Department of Food Science and Human Nutrition, Iowa State University, Ames, IA
**Robert M. Russell, M.D**. *(vice-chair),* Human Nutrition Research Center on Aging, Tufts University, Boston, MA
**Larry R. Beuchat, Ph.D.,** Center for Food Safety, University of Georgia, Griffin, GA
Susan Ference, D.V.M., Ph.D., SAF Risk, LC, Madison, WI
**Nancy F. Krebs, M.D.,** Department of Nutrition, University of Colorado Health Sciences Center, Denver, CO
**Shiriki Kumanyika, Ph.D.,** Center for Clinical Epidemiology and Biostatistics, University of Pennsylvania School of Medicine, Philadelphia, PA
**Reynaldo Martorell, Ph.D.,** Department of International Health, The Rollins School of Public Health, Emory University, Atlanta, GA
**Lynn Parker, M.S.**, Child Nutrition Programs and Nutrition Policy, Food Research and Action Center, Washington, DC
**Nicholas J. Schork, Ph.D.,** Department of Psychiatry, University of California, San Diego
**John W. Suttie, Ph.D.,** Department of Biochemistry, University of Wisconsin, Madison, WI
**Steve L. Taylor, Ph.D.**, Department of Food Science and Technology and Food Processing Center, University of Nebraska- Lincoln, Lincoln, NE
**Barry Zoumas, Ph.D.**, Department of Agricultural Economics and Rural Sociology, Pennsylvania State University, University Park, PA

The number of members can change from time to time. Each member serves for a term of up to three years. About one-third of the membership is replaced each year. Membership is generally limited to two terms.

## Declaration of Interests

The financial interests and connections of this RDA committee are held in confidence and not made public. We are assured by Dr Linda Meyers that checks on the suitability of the board members are made, but such information is kept confidential. The reader may consider this less than completely reassuring, given the extent of the disclosed financial connections to the pharmaceutical industry by the UK committee.

# Appendix D

## 101 problems with the RDA

A few of the major problems with the ascorbate RDA are:

1.  The RDA committee limited their considerations to doses below 200mg per day, discounting evidence relating to higher doses.
2.  The central NIH pharmacokinetic papers are invalid.
3.  The NIH sample size for young, adult, male subjects was seven. (The later study on females used 15 subjects.)
4.  The NIH redefined the word "saturation" to mean baseline level, causing all kinds of confusion among people who took it to mean chemical saturation.
5.  The committee did not recognise the problems with the NIH papers.
6.  The committee did not understand that the NIH choice of white blood cells was because they were easy to sample, rather than any biological merit.
7.  The committee incorrectly suggested that the NIH studies were "rigorous" and "unique".
8.  The committee did not use anything resembling a cost-benefit analysis, hence their analysis was biased.
9.  The committee did not provide any explanation for their use of the body pool as a measure of requirements.
10. No explanation was provided for the use of a static saturation measure, such as the body pool, for a dynamic and changeable physiology.
11. There was no explanation for why the committee assumed tissue saturation is physiologically more important than the maximum plasma steady state value.
12. No valid explanation was given for the use of white blood cells as a model for body tissues.
13. No explanation was given for the selection of neutrophils over other white blood cell types.
14. There was no valid explanation for the choice of white blood cells as opposed to red blood cells. Both are easy to sample.

15. No explanation of how neutrophils model general body tissues was provided.
16. No explanation was given for how neutrophils are "best", and the meaning of the term "best" was not specified.
17. There was no explanation of why, if they have the same absorption characteristics as normal body tissues, neutrophils contain so much ascorbate.
18. The committee did not do the simple calculation of what the body pool would be if body tissues behaved like neutrophils.
19. No discussion was provided of the relative concentration of ascorbate receptors in different body tissues.
20. There was no explanation of how the ascorbate transporters in neutrophils make them suitable as a model for other tissues.
21. There was no discussion of how representative neutrophil transporters are of those in other tissues.
22. No consideration was given to the fact that neutrophils absorb ascorbate more rapidly than most body tissues.
23. No consideration was given to the fact that neutrophils deplete more slowly than other body tissues.
24. There was no explanation of why neutrophil activation does not separate their requirements from other body tissues.
25. There was no explanation for the use of phagocytic cells as models for normal body tissues, which are not phagocytic.
26. There was no explanation of how neutrophil production of superoxide, hydrogen peroxide and other reactive species relates to normal body tissues.
27. There was no explanation for considering neutrophils to be independent of plasma ascorbate levels, when their production of and damage by superoxide is proportional to the plasma concentration, up to the maximum steady state value.
28. The committee selected neutrophil saturation as a measure, and then chose a lower value, based on excretion.
29. The low dose saturation of white blood cells (100mg intake), selected for the RDA, is only half a percent of the steady state limit in plasma (intakes of about 20 grams).

30. There was no explanation of how the committee could believe that the erroneous NIH studies measured steady state levels for plasma.
31. The committee did not explain their belief that ascorbate intakes above 200mg have little effect on plasma levels.
32. There was no explanation for believing the half-life of ascorbate is of the order of weeks.
33. The committee failed to understand the two-phase nature of ascorbate in plasma.
34. The NIH's bioavailability ideas are incorrect, because of the short half-life of vitamin C.
35. There was no appreciation of the fact that two 200mg doses taken 12 hours apart have the same absorption characteristics (bioavailability) as a single 200mg dose.
36. The committee's belief that only low doses are absorbed biased their evaluation of the data.
37. The committee did not mention the theory that heart disease is a result of prolonged ascorbate deficiency.
38. There was no mention of the physiology of other mammals, which synthesise ascorbate.
39. There was no explanation for their conclusion that people require only a small fraction of the dose needed in animals.
40. There was no explanation of why humans should not excrete ascorbate, when other animals excrete it.
41. The committee provided no explanation of why they thought excreted ascorbate was simply wasted. (This is NOT obvious, unless you are ignorant of physiological principles and drug action).
42. The committee did not explain that their Tolerable Upper Limit relies on the same mechanism as Cathcart's bowel tolerance method, but is cruder and less specific to the individual.
43. The Tolerable Upper Limit, if applied to healthy individuals, would permit high intakes in the range suggested by others (up to 20 grams).
44. There was no mention of the well-known increase in bowel tolerance during stress or illness.
45. The committee did not discuss the implications of greatly increased absorption during stress or illness.

46. The Tolerable Upper Limit depended on uncertainty (or fudge) factors – the source of these was not made clear.
47. 10% variation was assumed in the requirements of the human population in calculating the RDA – no explanation was given.
48. There is no explanation of how the RDA value encompasses 97-98% of the requirements for the population.
49. There was no explanation for the assumption that the nutritional range contains only low intakes.
50. Beneficial effects of high doses were seen as pharmacological rather than nutritional, but there was no explanation of this distinction.
51. There was no explanation of why observed beneficial effects of apparently safe high doses should be ignored, on the grounds that some studies did not show the effect.
52. A substance with a short half-life cannot be expected to achieve consistent results in studies that give only one dose per day; this was not explained or even mentioned.
53. There is no obvious mechanism for modifying the RDA recommendation in response to new scientific data.
54. The committee are unwilling or unable to provide a scientific defence of their recommendations.
55. The committee insisted on "compelling evidence" for high dose benefits, even though the toxicity is minimal.
56. The committee insisted on "consistent" positive data for high dose benefits, even though the toxicity is minimal.
57. The demand that studies showing benefits of a safe, high dose of ascorbate should be conclusive, despite minimal toxicity and low cost is incorrect.
58. The committee treated lack of response as a negative finding for high dose studies, despite minimal toxicity.
59. The suggestion that high dose benefits were not specific enough requires explanation.
60. It was not shown that scurvy is the only deficiency disease associated with ascorbate.
61. It was not shown that all deficiency diseases require ascorbate in micronutrient quantities.
62. Higher doses of ascorbate were not shown to be toxic.
63. It was not shown that measures of "good health" are at a maximum with low intakes.

64. It was not demonstrated that higher doses are in any way deleterious.
65. It was not established that people or vitamin C dependent animals are more resistant to stress at low intakes.
66. It was not shown that people or vitamin C dependent animals are more resistant to infection at low intakes.
67. It was not established that people or vitamin C dependent animals are more resistant to degenerative disease at low intakes.
68. No evidence was provided that animals that synthesise ascorbate produce only small amounts.
69. It was not shown that people are in optimal redox balance at low intakes.
70. The competing high dose hypothesis was not refuted.
71. There was no appreciation of the general equivalence of doses of 500mg and above, in healthy people.
72. References to the proposed benefits or to studies purporting to show large benefits for high-dose ascorbate were not included.
73. There was a general bias against high doses.
74. Amounts of ascorbate available from certain diets, such as the vegetarian diet, were underestimated.
75. Data from low dose studies were used in statements that implied future research should be limited to low doses.
76. Low doses were incorrectly stated to be optimal for heart disease.
77. The level of ascorbate catabolism or breakdown is not an indication of intake requirements.
78. Saturation was not defined, adding to the confusion caused by the NIH's redefinition of the term.
79. Little information was presented on the variation in requirements in the population.
80. It is quite possible that doses of several times the RDA will protect against serious disease; this possibility was ignored.
81. Many ascorbate transporters are really glucose transporters (GLUT), but the committee did not discuss the impact of glucose levels.
82. The number and expression of ascorbate transporters can be affected by factors such as insulin; this was not discussed.

83. The committee did not consider the health risks involved in underestimating the RDA.
84. RDA levels of ascorbate could be the cause of atherosclerosis.
85. RDA levels of ascorbate could be the cause of stroke.
86. RDA levels of ascorbate could be the leading cause of arthritis.
87. RDA levels of ascorbate could be a cause of degenerative brain disease.
88. RDA levels of ascorbate could reduce life expectancy.
89. The committee failed to show that deficiency diseases would not occur at their recommended intake.
90. The difference between nutritional effects and pharmacology was confused.
91. It was not shown that RDA level doses are safer than gram level doses.
92. There was no explanation of the biological implications of the loss of the ability to synthesise ascorbate in humans.
93. The evidence that some members of the population may retain a limited ability to manufacture ascorbate in the body was ignored.
94. There was no mention of alternative interpretations of the data.
95. Possible changes in human biochemistry, since the loss of our ability to synthesize ascorbate, were not considered.
96. There was no explanation of the likely effects of synthesis of ascorbate on survival value in animals, especially with reference to starvation.
97. No account of why most animals and plants have high levels of ascorbate was given.
98. The recommended intake of ascorbate in our nearest primate relatives was not considered in terms of comparative physiology.
99. There was no appreciation that studies of supplemental ascorbate show effects from doses far in excess of the supposed "saturated" values.
100. The synergy between ascorbate and other antioxidants was excluded.
101. We could have continued but decided to stop here.

Readers are invited to add to this list, email your contribution to radicalascorbate@yahoo.com.

# Appendix E

Here we will place valid evidence provided by the RDA committees, or other interested scientists, who have provided additional evidence in support of the RDA, its methods or background science. In particular, if the arguments in this book are shown to be invalid, we will report the new evidence here.

Dear Dr. Hickey.

While I thank you for the offer to respond in an appendix, as a matter of procedure the Institute of Medicine speaks only through its reports and does not provide "real time advice" or reactions independent of the reports.

Thus, we decline your offer.

Linda D. Meyers, Ph.D.
Director, Food and Nutrition Board
Institute of Medicine
National Academies
500 Fifth Street, NW
Washington, DC 20001

Dear Dr. Hickey and Mr. Sardi:

Your respective e-mail communications of February 13 and 14, 2005 to Dr. Zerhouni, Director, National Institutes of Health (NIH), concerning scientific information on the topic of vitamin C has been shared with and reviewed by representatives of several NIH Institutes, Centers, and Offices. I have been asked to provide a collective response on behalf of NIH.

As you know and has been stated in a prior communication related to your concerns, the NIH does not determine the RDAs; rather, they have been set by the Food and Nutrition Board of the Institute of Medicine/National Academy of Sciences. As stated in the published Dietary Reference Intakes for Vitamin C, Vitamin E, Selenium, and Carotenoids (IOM, 2000), the RDAs for vitamin C are based on an intake of vitamin C that maintains near-maximal neutrophil vitamin C concentrations with minimal urinary loss. RDAs for vitamin C are not based on the saturation of plasma. We have been in communication with the staff of the Food and Nutrition Board to make them aware of your concerns.

As you are aware, biomedical scientific investigations hopefully lead to new information on which to ultimately build recommendations for improved health. In making these recommendations, the data in the peer-reviewed literature are taken collectively and are evaluated by various groups so that the best possible recommendations emerge. The publications that you cite are of interest, but by themselves do not directly indicate that misinformation is being communicated.

Again, your longstanding interest in the RDA for vitamin C is appreciated and your concerns have been noted. We expect that future research will provide us with information to make appropriate modifications to the current recommendations for improved health and prevention of disease.

Sincerely,
Van S. Hubbard, M.D., Ph.D.
CAPT, USPHS
Director, NIH Division of Nutrition Research Coordination
National Institutes of Health,
Department of Health and Human Services
Two Democracy Plaza, Room 631,
6707 Democracy Boulevard MSC 5461
Bethesda, Maryland 20892-5461

Readers will be able to judge for themselves if these responses refute our objections to the low dose recommendations for vitamin C. Over 2000 copies of this book were made freely available for download from the Internet, for scientists, physicians, nutritionists and members of the public to review. This was the most demanding form of peer review. No objection to the science presented has been communicated to the authors.

# Glossary

**Antioxidant**: Any chemical or action that prevents oxidation.

**Arteriole**: A small artery.

**Ascorbate**: An alternative name for vitamin C.

**Ascorbic acid**: An alternative name for vitamin C.

**Ascorbyl radical**: An oxidised form of ascorbate which has donated a single electron. The ascorbyl radical lies between ascorbate and dehydroascorbate.

**Atherosclerosis**: Damage and thickening to the blood vessel wall.

**Bioavailability**: A misleading term for relative absorption.

**Biomarker**: A measurement associated with a biological function.

**Blastogenesis**: When a cell multiplies by simple division or budding.

**Bowel tolerance**: A measure of the vitamin C requirements for an individual, after Dr Robert Cathcart.

**Catalyst**: A substance that increases the rate of a chemical reaction without being consumed in the reaction.

**Cataract**: Clouding of the lens of the eye.

**Chemotaxis**: Movement of the cell towards a chemical stimulus.

**Colorectal**: Pertaining to or involving the colon or rectum.

**Decision theory**: A body of knowledge and related mathematical techniques developed from the fields of statistics, mathematics, and logic designed to aid in making decisions under conditions of uncertainty.

**Dehydroascorbate**: A doubly oxidised form of vitamin C (ascorbate).

**Dermal**: Pertaining to the skin.

**Dynamic flow**: The intake of ascorbate that produces a continuous flow through the tissues with a reserve in the gut.

**Enzyme**: A protein (or possibly RNA) that catalyses a chemical reaction.

**Epinephrine**: Another name for adrenaline. A hormone secreted by the adrenal gland which increases blood pressure, heart rate and cardiac output.

**Free radical**: A molecule with at least one unpaired electron. Free radicals are highly reactive and react rapidly with other molecules, disrupting normal cellular processes, causing cellular damage and oxidative stress.

**Game theory**: Game theory is similar to decision theory. A major difference between the two is that in game theory the decision is being made vis-à-vis an opponent, whereas in decision theory the only opponent is "nature" with its related uncertainty.

**Gastritis**: Inflammation of the lining of the stomach.

**Glucose-6-phosphatase**: An enzyme involved in the metabolism of glucose.

**Glucuronidase**: An enzyme involved in metabolism.

**GLUT**: A glucose transporter, some forms of which will also pump dehydroascorbate.

**Glutathione**: An antioxidant normally found in most cells.

**Haemochromatosis**: A disorder of iron metabolism characterized by excessive absorption.

**Hyperaemia**: increased blood in an organ or tissue.

**Hypothesis**: An idea to be tested by scientific experiment.

**Heuristic**: Rule of thumb.

**Insulin**: A hormone that regulates blood glucose.

**In vitro**: Within glass, a test tube experiment.

**In vivo**: Within the body or organism.

**LDL**: Low density lipoprotein is a particle used to transport cholesterol.

**Lipid**: An oil or fat.

**Lymphocyte**: A white blood cell.

**Neutrophil**: A white blood cell specialised for phagocytosis.

**Micro-aneurysm**: A swelling that forms on the side of tiny blood vessels, which may burst and bleed into nearby tissue. Often found in the retina of the eye in people with diabetes.

**Micromole**: A measurement of concentration, 1/1000 of a millimole.

**Millimole**: A measurement of concentration, 1/1000 of a mole.

**Mole**: The molecular weight of a substance expressed in grams, or a small furry creature. Here used as a measure of concentration where one mole of substance ($6.023 \times 10^{23}$ molecules) is dissolved in one litre of solution.

**Monocyte**: A large phagocytic white blood cell.

**Myeloperoxidase**: An enzyme involved in killing bacteria.

**Optimal**: Most favourable or desirable, a mechanism which results in the greatest net gain for the specified action.

**Oxidation**: Rapid chemical reaction similar to burning, which involves loss of an electron or a hydrogen nucleus (proton) from a molecule.

**Paradigm**: A model, theory or belief.

**Peroxidation**: In this context, the process by which fatty acids get oxidized.

**Pericorneal**: Surrounding the cornea.

**Phagocyte**: A cell that eats or engulfs foreign bodies.

**Pharmacokinetics**: Science of movement of drugs in the body.

**Pharmacology**: Science of drugs.

**Plasma**: Fluid surrounding or containing cells.

**Polyp**: Structure consisting of a rounded head, which grows outward from a broad base or stalk.

**Probability**: a number between 0 and 1 which represents how likely some event is to occur. A probability of 0 means the event will never occur, while a probability of 1 means that the event will always occur.

**RDA**: A biased nutritional recommendation, based on politics or a government figure based on rigorous science (reader to decide).

**Receptor**: A molecule, on the surface of a cell, that binds with drugs, antigens, antibodies or other cellular or immunological components.

**Redox**: Pertaining to reduction and oxidation.

**Reduction**: Gain of electrons or hydrogen atoms (protons) by a molecule.

**Risk**: A quantitative or qualitative expression of possible loss, which considers the probability that a hazard will cause harm and the resulting consequences.

**Standard deviation**: A statistical measure of variation.

**Steady state**: Condition of a body or system in which the conditions at each point do not change with time, after initial fluctuations have disappeared.

**Substrate**: A substance acted upon by an enzyme.

**SVCT**: Sodium dependent vitamin C transporter, which pumps ascorbate.

**Toxic**: Poisonous.

**Transporter**: A molecular pump found in the membranes of cells.

**Vasculature**: Blood vessels.

**Venule**: A small vein.

**White blood cells**: Specialised cells of the immune system found in the blood.

# The original book

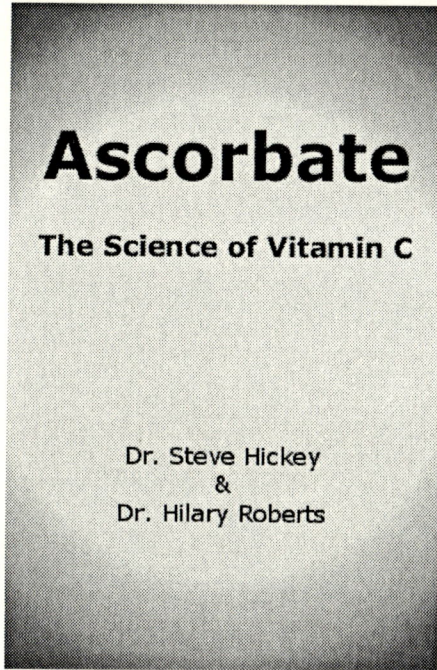

## Ascorbate

### The Science of Vitamin C

Dr. Steve Hickey
&
Dr. Hilary Roberts

## Comments on Ascorbate:

"...a truly fantastic book" Dr Selva Kumar

"Utterly honest, easy to understand, *Ascorbate, The Science of Vitamin C* is a real treasure." Professor Joel Kaufman

"This is an historic book, one that will be treasured by those who embrace natural health approaches and a revelation to the uninformed." Bill Sardi

# References

[1] Expert Group on Vitamins and Minerals (1999), UK government update paper EVM/99/21/P.

[2] EVM (2002) Revised review of vitamin C, UK government publication, EVM/99/21.

[3] EVM (2003) Safe upper limits for vitamins and minerals, UK Government publication.

[4] EVM (2003) Review of vitamin C, UK Government publication.

[5] Committee on Medical Aspects of Food Policy (1991) Dietary Reference Values for Food Energy and Nutrients for the United Kingdom. Report on Health and Social Subjects, No. 41, HMSO, London.

[6] Burns L. (2004) UK Food Standards Agency, personal communication to Dr Hickey.

[7] Food and Nutrition Board (RDA Committee) (1992) Recommended Dietary Allowances (Dietary Reference Intakes), 10th edition, National Academy Press.

[8] RDA Committee (2000) Dietary Reference Intakes for Vitamin C, Selenium and Carotenoids, The National Academy of Science, United States.

[9] Hickey S. Roberts H. (2004) Ascorbate, The Science of Vitamin C, Lulu Press.

[10] Pauling L. (1986) How to live longer and feel better, Avon Books, New York.

[11] Levy T.E. (2002) Vitamin C, Infectious Disease and Toxins, Xlibris, Philadelphia.

[12] Chernoff H. Moses L. (1987) Elementary Decision Theory, Dover, Publications, New York.

[13] Kaplan M. (1998) Decision Theory as Philosophy, reprint edition, Cambridge University Press, England.

[14] Williams R.J. (1998) Biochemical Individuality: The Basis for the Genetotrophic Concept, Keats Publishing, Connecticut.

[15] Levine M. Conry-Cantilena C. Wang Y. Welch R. W. Phillip W. Washko P.W. Dhariwal K.R. Park J.B. Lazarrev A. Graumlich J.F. King J. Cantilena L.R. (1996) Vitamin C pharmacokinetics in healthy volunteers: Evidence for a recommended dietary allowance, Proc. Natl. Acad. Sci. USA, 93, 3704–3709.

[16] Cameron E. Campbell A. (1991) Innovation vs. quality control: an 'unpublishable' clinical trial of supplemental ascorbate in incurable cancer, Medical Hypotheses, 36(3), 185-189.

[17] Levine M. Wang Y. Padayatty S.J. Morrow J. (2001) A new recommended dietary allowance of vitamin C for healthy young women Proc. Natl. Acad. Sci. USA, 14, 98 (17), 9842-9846.

[18] von Neumann J. Morgenstern O. (1944), Theory of Games and Economic Behavior, Princeton University Press, USA.

[19] Osbourne M.J. (2003) An Introduction to Game Theory, Oxford University Press, England.

[20] Nash J.F. Nash J.F jr (1997) Essays on Game Theory, Edward Elgar Publishing, Cheltenham, England.

[21] Layard R. Glaister S. (1994) Cost-Benefit Analysis, second edition, Cambridge University Press, England.

[22] Gigerenzer G. (2002) Calculated Risks, Simon and Shuster, New York.

[23] Scientific Advisory Committee on Nutrition (2002) Paper for discussion: A Framework for Evaluation of Evidence that Relates Food and Nutrients to Health, Agenda Item, 520/06/02 SACN/02/02A.

[24] Scientific Advisory Committee on Nutrition (2004) Advice of fish consumption: benefits and risks, TSO, London.

[25] Sheen C.L. Dillon J.F. Bateman D.N. Simpson K.J. MacDonald T.M. (2002) Paracetamol-related deaths in Scotland 1994-2000, British Journal of Clinical Pharmacology, 54, 430.

[26] Atcha Z. (2000) Paracetamol related deaths in England and Wales 1993 – 1997, Health Statistics Quarterly, 7, 59.

[27] Editorial (1996) Reducing paracetamol overdoses, BMJ, 313, 1417-1418.

[28] Price K.D. Price C.S. Reynolds R.D. (1996) Hyperglycemia-induced latent scurvy and atherosclerosis: the scorbutic-metaplasia hypothesis, Med Hypotheses, 46(2), 119-129.

[29] Clemetson C.A. (1999) The key role of histamine in the development of atherosclerosis and coronary heart disease, Med Hypotheses, 52(1), 1-8.

[30] Rath M. Pauling L. (1989) Unified Theory of Human Cardiovascular Disease Leading the Way to the Abolition of this Disease as a Cause for Human Mortality, Arteriosclerosis, 9, 579-592.

[31] Cheraskin E. Ringsdorf W.M. Sisley E.L. (1983) The Vitamin C Connection, Harper and Row, New York.

[32] Levine M. Rumsey S. Wang Y. Park J. Kwon O. Xu W. Amano N. (1996) Vitamin C, In Ziegler E.E. Filer J.J. Present Knowledge in Nutrition, 7th Ed. Washington, DC, ISLI Press, 146-159.

[33] Henning S.M. Zhang J.Z. McKee R.W. SwenSeid M.E. Jacob R.A. (1991) Glutathione blood levels and other antioxidant defence indices in men fed diets low in vitamin C, C.J.Nutrition,121, 1969-1975.

[34] Baker E.M. Hodges R.E. Hood J. Sauberlich H.E. March S.C. Canham J.E. (1971) Metabolism of $C_{14}$ and $H_3$ labelled L-ascorbic acid in human scurvy, American Journal of Clinical Nutrition, 24, 444-454.

[35] Kallner A. Hartmann I. Hornig D. (1979) Steady-state turnover and body pool of ascorbic acid in man, American Journal of Clinical Nutrition, 32, 530-539.

[36] Olson J.A. and Hodges R.E. (1987) Recommended dietary intakes (RDI) of vitamin C in humans. American Journal of Clinical Nutrition, 45, 693-703.

[37] Kallner, A. et al (1981) On the requirements of ascorbic acid in man: steady-state turnover and body pool in smokers. American Journal of Clinical Nutrition, 34, 1347-1355.

[38] Lewin S. (1976) Vitamin C: Its Molecular Biology and Medical Potential, Academic Press.

[39] Omaye S.T. Schous E.E. Kutnink M.A. Hawkes W.C. (1987) Measurement of vitamin C in blood components by high performance liquid chromatography, implications in assessing vitamin C status, Ann NY Acad Sci, 498, 389-401.

[40] Wei-Jun L. Johnson D. Jarvis S.M. (2001) Vitamin C transport systems of mammalian cells, Molecular Membrane Biology, 18(1), 87-95.

[41] Washko P. Levine M.J. (1992) Inhibition of ascorbic acid transport in human neutrophils by glucose, Biol Chem, 267(33), 23568-23574.

[42] Olson A.L. Pessin J.E. (1996) Structure, function and regulation of the mammalian facilitative glucose transporter gene family, Annu Rev Nutr, 16, 235-256.

[43] Mueckler M. (1994) Facilitative glucose transporters, Eur J Biochem, 219, 713-725.

[44] Santisteban G.A., Ely J.T. (1985) Glycemic modulation of tumor tolerance in a mouse model of breast cancer, Biochem Biophys Res Commun, 132(3), 1174-1179.

[45] Hamel E.E. Santisteban G.A. Ely J.T. Read D.H. (1986) Hyperglycemia and reproductive defects in non-diabetic gravidas: a mouse model test of a new theory, Life Sci , 39(16), 1425-1428.

[46] Ely J.T. (1996) Glycemic Modulation of Tumor Tolerance, J Orthomolecular Med, 11(1), 23-34.

[47] Fladeby C. Skar R. Serck-Hanssen G. (2003) Distinct regulation of glucose transport and GLUT1/GLUT3 transporters by glucose deprivation and IGF-I in chromaffin cells, Biochim Biophys Acta, 17, 1593(2-3), 201-208.

[48] Stone I. (1974) The Healing Factor: Vitamin C Against Disease, Putnam, New York.

[49] Cathcart R.F. (1981) Vitamin C titrating to bowel tolerance, anascorbemia and acute induced scurvy, Medical Hypotheses, 7, 1359-1376.

[50] Padayatty S.J. Sun H. Wang Y. Riordan H.D. Hewitt S.M. Katz A. Wesley R.A. Levine M. (2004) Vitamin C pharmacokinetics: implications for oral and intravenous use, Ann Intern Med, 140(7), 533-537.

[51] Rose S. Bullock S. (1991) The Chemistry of Life, Penquin Books, London.

[52] Daruwala R. Song J. Koh W.S. Rumsey S.C. Levine M. (1999) Cloning and functional characterization of the human sodium-dependent vitamin C transporters hSVCT1 and hSVCT2, FEBS Lett, 5, 460(3), 480-484.

[53] Levine M. (2004) Personal communication.

[54] Benke K.K. (1999) Modelling Ascorbic Acid Level in Plasma and Its Dependence on Absorbed Dose, Journal of the Australasian College of Nutritional & Environmental Medicine, 18(1), 11-12.

[55] Padayatty S.J. Sun H. Wang Y. Riordan H.D. Hewitt S.M. Katz A. Wesley R.A. Levine M. (2004) Vitamin C pharmacokinetics: implications for oral and intravenous use, Ann Intern Med, 140(7), 533-537.

[56] Baker E.M. et al (1969) Metabolism of ascorbic-1-14C acid in experimental human Scurvy, American Journal of Clinical Nutrition, 22(5), 549-558.

[57] Kallner, A. et al (1977) On the absorption of ascorbic acid in man. International Journal of Vitamin and Nutrition Research, 47, 383-388.

[58] Goldstein A. Aronow L. Kalman S.M. (1974) Principles of Drug Action, John Wiley and Sons, New York.

[59] Cathcart R.F. (1985) Vitamin C: nhe nontoxic, nonrate-limited, antioxidant free radical scavenger, Medical Hypotheses, 18, 61-77.

[60] Shiu-Ming K. MacLean M.E. McCormick K. Wilson J.X. (2004) Gender and sodium-ascorbate transporter isoforms determine ascorbate concentrations in Mice, J. Nutr., 134, 2216-2221.

[61] Ely J.T. (1999) Ascorbic Acid and Some Other Modern Analogs of the Germ Theory Journal of Orthomolecular Medicine, 14 (3), 143-56.

[62] Wang H. Dutta B. Huang W. Devoe L.D. Leibach F.H. Ganapathy V. Prasad P.D. (1999) Human Na(+)-dependent vitamin C transporter 1 (hSVCT1): primary structure,

functional characteristics and evidence for a non-functional splice variant, Biochim Biophys Acta, 9, 1461(1), 1-9.

[63] FDA (1998) Substances generally recognised as safe, Code of Federal Regulations, title 21 - Food and Drugs, Vol 3, Parts 170 to 199, U.S. Government Printing Office, 437.

[64] Levine M. Rumsey S.C. Daruwala R. Park J.B. Wang Y. (1999) Criteria and recommendations for vitamin C intake, JAMA, 281, 1415–1423.

[65] Johnston C.S. Cox S.K. (2001) Plasma-Saturating Intakes of Vitamin C Confer Maximal Antioxidant Protection to Plasma, J Am Col Nutrition, 20(6), 623-627.

[66] Halliwell B. and Gutteridge J.M.C. (1999) Free Radicals in Biology and Medicine, OUP, Oxford, England.

[67] Kojo S. (2004) Vitamin C: basic metabolism and its function as an index of oxidative stress, Curr Med Chem, 11(8), 1041-1064.

[68] Denno R. Takabayashi A. Sugano M. Awane M. Jin M.B. Morimoto T. Tanaka K. Yamaoka Y. Kobayashi N. Ozawa K.J. (1995) The ratio of reduced glutathione/oxidized glutathione is maintained in the liver during short-term hepatic hypoxia, Gastroenterol, 30(3), 338-346.

[69] Buettner G.R. (1993) The pecking order of free radicals and antioxidants, Lipid peroxidation, a-tocopherol, and ascorbate, Arch Biochem Biophy, 300, 535-543.

[70] Anderson R. Lukey P.T. (1987) A biological role for ascorbate in selective neutralisation of extracellular phagocyte derived oxidants, Ann NY Acad Sci, 498, 229-247.

[71] Halliwell B. Wasil M. Grootveld M. (1987) Biologically significant scavenging of the myeloperoxidase derived oxidant hypochlorous acid by ascorbic acid, Febs Lett, 213, 15-17.

[72] Washko P. Rotrosen D. Levine M. (1989) Ascorbic acid transport and accumulation in human neutrophils, J Biol Chem, 264(32), 18996-19002.

[73] Welch R.W. Wang Y. Crossman A. Jr. Park J.B. Kirk K.L. Levine M. (1995) Accumulation of vitamin C (ascorbate) and its oxidized metabolite dehydroascorbic acid occurs by separate mechanisms, J Biol Chem, 270(21), 12584-12592.

[74] Wang Y. Russo T.A. Kwon O. Chanock S. Rumsey S.C. Levine M. (1997) Ascorbate recycling in human neutrophils: Induction by bacteria, Proc Natl Acad Sci U S A, 94(25), 13816–13819.

[75] Washko P. Yang Y. Levine M. (1993) Ascorbic acid recycling in human neutrophils, J Biol Chem, 268(21), 15531-15535.

[76] Rumsey S.C. Kwon O. Xu G.W. Burant C.F. Simpson I. Levine M., (1997) Glucose transporter isoforms GLUT1 and GLUT3 transport dehydroascorbic acid, J Biol Chem., 272(30), 18982-18989.

[77] Levine M. (2002) Personal communication to Dr Hickey.

[78] Hornig D. Weber F. Wiss O. (1971) Uptake and release of [1-14C] ascorbic acid and [1-14C] dehydroascorbic acid by erythrocytes of guinea pigs, Clin Chim Acta, 31, 25-35.

[79] Hughes R.E. Maton S.C. (1968) The passage of vitamin C across the erythrocyte membrane, Brit J Haematol, 14, 247-253.

[80] Wagner E. White S.W. Jennings M. Bennett K. (1987) The entrapment of [14C] ascorbic acid in human Erythrocytes, Biochim Biophys Acta, 902, 133-136.

[81] Okamura M. (1979) Uptake of L-ascorbic acid and L-dehydroascorbic acid by human erythrocytes and HeLa cells, J Nutr Sci Vitaminol, 25, 269-279.

[82] Evans R.M. Currie L. Campbell A. (1982) The distribution of ascorbic acid between various cellular components of blood, in normal individuals, and its relation to the plasma concentration, Br J Nutr, 47, 473-482.

[83] May J.M. (1998) Ascorbate function and metabolism in the human erythrocyte, Frontiers in Bioscience, 2, 1-10.

[84] Wang Y. Russo T.A. Kwan O. Chanock S. Rumsey S.C. Levine M. (1997) Ascorbate recycling in human neutrophils: induction by bacteria, Proc Natl Acad Sci USA, 94, 13816-13819.

[85] Byun J. Mueller D.M. Fabjan J.S. Heinecke J.W. (1999) Nitrogen dioxide radical generated by the myeloperoxidase-hydrogen peroxide-nitrite system promotes lipid peroxidation of low density lipoprotein, FEBS Lett, 455(3), 243-246.

[86] Gey K.F. (1998) Vitamins E plus C and interacting nutrients required for optimal health. A critical and constructive review of epidemiology and supplementation data regarding cardiovascular disease and cancer, Biofactors, 7, 113-174.

[87] Rath M, Pauling L. (1991) Solution to the puzzle of human cardiovascular disease: Its primary cause is ascorbate deficiency, leading to the deposition of lipoprotein (a) and fibrinogen/fibrin in the vascular wall, Journal of Orthomolecular Medicine, 6, 125-134.

[88] Pauling L. Rath M. (1994) Prevention and treatment of occlusive cardiovascular disease with ascorbate and substances that inhibit the binding of lipoprotein (A), US patent 5, 278, 189.

[89] Lykkesfeldt J. Loft S. Neilsen J.B. Poulson I.I.E. (1997) Ascorbic acid and dehdroascorbic acid as biomarkers of oxidative stress caused by smoking, Am J Clin Nutr, 65, 959-963.

[90] Reilly M. Delanty N. Lawson J.A. Fitzgerald G.A. (1996) Modulation of oxidant stress in vivo in chronic cigarette smokers, Circulation, 94, 19-25.

[91] Panayiotidis M. Collins A.R. (1997) Ex vivo assessment of lymphocyte antioxidant status using the comet assay, Free Rad Research, 27, 533-537.

[92] Osganian S.K. Stampfer M.J. Rimm E. Spiegelman D. Hu F.B. Manson J.E. Willett W.C. (2003) Vitamin C and risk of coronary heart disease in women, J Am Coll Cardiol, 42(2), 246-252.

[93] Fletcher A.E. Breeze E. Shetty P.S. (2003) Antioxidant vitamins and mortality in older persons: findings from the nutrition add-on study to the Medical Research Council Trial of Assessment and Management of Older People in the Communit, Am J Clin Nutr, 78(5), 999-1010.

[94] Loria C.M. Klag M.J. Caulfield L.E. Whelton P.K. (2000) Vitamin C status and mortality in US adults, Am J Clin Nutr, 72(1), 139-145.

[95] Simon J.A. Hudes E.S. Browner W.S. (1998) Serum ascorbic acid and cardiovascular disease prevalence in U.S. adults, Epidemiology, 9(3), 316-321.

[96] Khaw K.T. Bingham S. Welch A. Luben R. Wareham N. Oakes S. Day N. (2001) Relation between plasma ascorbic acid and mortality in men and women in EPIC-Norfolk prospective study: a prospective population study. European Prospective Investigation into Cancer and Nutrition, Lancet, 357(9257), 657-663.

[97] Willis G.C. (1957) The reversibility of atheroslerosis, Canad. M. A. J., 77, 106-109.

[98] Willis G.C. Light A.W. Cow W.S. (1954) Serial arteriography in atherolsclerosis, Canad. M. A. J., 71, 562-568.

[99] Willis G.C. (1953) An experimental study of the intimal ground substance in atherosclerosis, Canad. M. A. J., 69, 17-22.

[100] Turley S.D. West C.E. Horton B.J. (1976) The role of ascorbic acid in the regulation of cholesterol metabolism and in the pathogenesis of artherosclerosis, Atherosclerosis, 24(1-2), 1-18.

[101] Knekt P. Ritz J. Pereira M.A. O'Reilly E.J. et al (2004) Antioxidant vitamins and coronary heart disease risk: a pooled analysis of 9 cohorts, American Journal of Clinical Nutrition, 80(6) 1508-1520.

[102] Marchioli R. Schweiger C. Levantesi G. Tavazzi L. Valagussa F. (2001) Antioxidant vitamins and prevention of cardiovascular disease: epidemiological and clinical trial data, Lipids, 36 Suppl, S53-63.

[103] Taylor C.A. Hampl J.S. Johnston C.S. (2000) Low intakes of vegetables and fruits, especially citrus fruits, lead to inadequate vitamin C intakes among adults, Eur J Clin Nutr, 54(7), 573-578.

[104] Hubbard L.D. Brothers R.J. King W.N. Clegg L.X. Klein R. Cooper L.S. Sharrett A.R. Davis M.D. (1999) Methods for evaluation of retinal microvascular abnormalities associated with hypertension/sclerosis in the Atherosclerosis Risk in Communities Study, Cai J.Ophthalmology, 106(12), 2269-2280.

[105] Klein R. Sharrett A.R. Klein B.E. Chambless L.E. Cooper L.S. Hubbard L.D. Evans G. (2000) Are retinal arteriolar abnormalities related to atherosclerosis?: The Atherosclerosis Risk in Communities Study, Arterioscler Thromb Vasc Biol, 20(6),1644-1650.

[106] Wong T.Y. Klein R. Couper D.J. Cooper L.S. Shahar E. Hubbard L.D. Wofford M.R. Sharrett A.R. (2001) Retinal microvascular abnormalities and incident stroke: the Atherosclerosis Risk in Communities Study, Lancet, 6, 358(9288), 1134-1140.

[107] Wong T.Y. Shankar A. Klein R. Klein B.E.K. Hubbard L.D. (2004) Prospective cohort study of retinal vessel diameters and risk of hypertension, BMJ, 329, 79.

[108] Wang J.J. Mitchell P. Leung H. Rochtchina E. Wong T.Y. Klein R. (2003) Hypertensive retinal vessel wall signs in a general older population, the blue mountains eye study, Hypertension, 42, 534-542.

[109] Wong T.Y. Klein R. Sharrett A.R. Duncan B.B. Couper D.J. Tielsch J.M. Klein B.E. Hubbard L.D. (2002) Retinal arteriolar narrowing and risk of coronary heart disease in men and women. The Atherosclerosis Risk in Communities Study, JAMA, 287(9), 1153-1159.

[110] Leung H. Wang J.J. Rochtchina E. Tan A.G. Wong T.Y. Klein R. Hubbard L.D. Mitchell P. (2003) Relationships between age, blood pressure, and retinal vessel diameters in an older population, Investigative Ophthalmology and Visual Science, 44, 2900-2904.

[111] Chiolero A. (2004) Arteriolar narrowing as predictor of hypertension: Blood pressure and weight gain are better, BMJ, 329, 514.

[112] Wong T. Shankar A. (2004) Arteriolar narrowing as predictor of hypertension: Authors' reply, BMJ, 329, 514-515.

[113] Bush S.J. (2004), CardioRetinometry, BMJ Rapid response, 23 July.

[114] Vermeera K.A. Vosa F.M. Lemijb H.G. Vossepoela A.M. (2004) A model based method for retinal blood vessel detection, Computers in Biology and Medicine, 34, 209–219.

[115] Hoover A. Kouznetsova V. Goldbaum M. (2000) Locating blood vessels in retinal images by piece-wise threshold probing of a matched filter response, IEEE Transactions on Medical Imaging, 19(3), 203-208.

[116] Gang L. Chutatape O. Krishnan S.M. (2002) Detection and measurement of retinal vessels in fundus images using amplitude modified second-order Gaussian filter, IEEE Trans Biomed Eng, 49(2), 168-172.

[117] Lalondey M. Gagnony L. Boucherz M. (2000) Non-recursive paired tracking for vessel extraction from retinal images, presented at the Conference Vision Interface 2000, Montréal.

[118] Couper D.J. Klein R. Hubbard L.D. Wong T.Y. Sorlie P.D. Cooper L.S. Brothers R.J. Nieto F.J. (2002) Reliability of retinal photography in the assessment of retinal microvascular characteristics: the Atherosclerosis Risk in Communities Study, Am J Ophthalmol, 133(1), 78-88.

Printed in the United States
39292LVS00007B/76-78

9 781411 622210